PRAISE FOR
HEAL THE HEALER

"A timely wake-up call along with practical strategies for preventing and recovering from burnout. . . . I highly recommend this book to the millions of healers worldwide seeking to recharge and continue their meaningful work without sacrificing their well-being. *Heal the Healer* provides a clear blueprint for sustaining passion, reigniting purpose, and making an even greater collective impact."

—DANIEL G. AMEN, MD, CEO and founder of Amen Clinics and author of *Change Your Brain, Change Your Life*

"If you are a healer feeling the strain of over-responsibility, this book is an invaluable resource. Joshua explores the roots of healer tendencies like self-sacrifice. He guides readers to heal old wounds and establish boundaries while emphasizing the power of coming together as a community."

—LYNDA CLOUD, CEO of the Institute for Integrative Nutrition and Chopra Education

"*Heal the Healer* is not just a book; it's a testament to the resilience and dedication of those who dedicate their lives to healing, reminding us that in order to change our world, we must first learn to change ourselves."

—MIKE HOFFMAN, founder and chairman emeritus of Changing Our World

"We can't give from an empty cup. Joshua has found a way to help healers understand the importance of taking care of themselves so they can make an even greater impact on the lives of others."

—ALEX ANZALONE, author, futurist, and Integrative Nutrition Health Coach

HEAL THE HEALER

HEAL THE HEALER

A SELF-CARE GUIDE for WELLNESS WORKERS and CAREGIVERS

Joshua Rosenthal

W

WONDERWELL

While every effort has been made to ensure the accuracy of the information in this book, it is intended for general guidance only. The author and publisher do not assume liability for any errors, inaccuracies, omissions, inconsistencies, or consequences arising from the use of this information.

This book should not be used as a substitute for professional, medical, psychological, or legal advice. Readers are encouraged to use their discretion when applying the principles, techniques, or recommendations presented in this book to their own lives. The author and publisher do not guarantee specific results or outcomes, and individual experiences may vary.

Published by Wonderwell Press
Austin, TX
www.rivergrovebooks.com

This work is being published under the Wonderwell Press imprint by an exclusive arrangement with Wonderwell. Wonderwell, Wonderwell Press, and the Wonderwell logos are wholly-owned trademarks of Wonderwell.

Distributed by River Grove Books

Design and composition by Adrian Morgan
Cover design by Adrain Morgan
Cover images used under license from ©Shutterstock.com

Publisher's Cataloging-in-Publication data is available.

Print ISBN: 978-1-963827-39-2

eBook ISBN: 978-1-63756-054-9

First Edition

In loving memory of my parents,
Valerie and Arthur

CONTENTS

FOREWORD

A S BOTH A PSYCHIATRIST AND BRAIN imaging specialist, I have dedicated my career to understanding how our brains influence every aspect of our lives. My research using SPECT imaging to analyze brain activity has shown me time and again that toxic stress damages the brain. When we are overworked, under slept, and emotionally depleted, our prefrontal cortex doesn't function properly. We lose access to our higher cognitive skills like focus, judgment, and empathy.

This is precisely why we are facing an epidemic of healer burnout. As doctors, nurses, therapists, social workers, caregivers, and other healers strive heroically to meet swelling care needs, they are spread dangerously thin. They contend with tremendous stress that often goes unacknowledged. The global trauma of the COVID-19 pandemic has only amplified this crisis, leaving many healers traumatized themselves.

As healers, we pour ourselves into helping others, frequently neglecting our own needs in the process. We operate in constant high-alert mode, absorbing others' trauma. No wonder so many of us suffer from exhaustion, anxiety, brain fog, and compassion fatigue. Our brains desperately need respite. Without proper rest and recovery, we cannot sustain the compassionate care of others.

That's why I was thrilled to receive an advance copy of Joshua Rosenthal's essential new book, *Heal the Healer*. As the pioneering founder of the Institute for Integrative Nutrition, Joshua understands firsthand the unique demands faced by those working in helping professions today. In this book, he provides a timely wake-up call along with practical strategies for preventing and recovering from burnout.

Drawing on decades of experience mentoring healers, Joshua compellingly illustrates how self-sacrifice and blurred work-life boundaries put us at risk. He explains the personality traits and childhood wounds that can predispose certain caring people to overfunction and ignore self-care needs. Importantly, he emphasizes that we can rewrite limiting beliefs and behaviors stemming from social conditioning and trauma. Through thoughtful exercises focused on clarifying values, setting boundaries, and envisioning an ideal future self, Joshua guides readers to reclaim their power.

Heal the Healer makes the crucial point that we need community to thrive. As Joshua writes, "When we have the support of a loving community, we are stronger." By coming together and exchanging wisdom, empathy, and resources, we can lift each other up. No healer needs to weather life's storms alone. Support allows us to process collective trauma, grieve, restore depleted reserves, and gain strength in numbers.

I highly recommend this book to the millions of healers worldwide seeking to recharge and continue their meaningful work without sacrificing their well-being. *Heal the Healer* provides a clear blueprint for sustaining passion, reigniting purpose, and making an even greater collective impact. This book arrives at a pivotal cultural moment, when burnout threatens our healthcare and helping systems. By supporting healers and caregivers, we safeguard access to compassionate care while catalyzing societal healing.

DANIEL G. AMEN, MD
CEO and founder of Amen Clinics and author of *Change Your Brain, Change Your Life*

PREFACE

WHEN THE PANDEMIC WAS AT ITS PEAK and healthcare workers were struggling with extreme stress, Joshua came up with the idea to write a book called *Heal the Healer*. It was a crucial question that needed to be answered: Who takes care of those who take care of others? Joshua's words struck a chord. Healers are everywhere, from medical professionals to caregivers, teachers, coaches, and counselors. Their services are in high demand. And many are so focused on helping others that they forget to take care of themselves, leading to exhaustion and a lack of joy in life. As Joshua points out, healers need healing, too.

When I first met Joshua fourteen years ago, he was deeply involved with the Institute for Integrative Nutrition. I watched him work tirelessly as director of the school while increasingly struggling with his own health. On one hand, his strong will and dedication helped him move mountains. On the other hand, his health and happiness suffered. Since that time, slowly but surely, he has been able to turn toward areas of his life that needed healing and attention. Learning to better care for himself has been a crucial part of Joshua's journey and has inspired him to guide others in this area.

As a healer myself, I understand the detrimental effects of unconsciously overgiving, self-sacrificing, and not setting proper boundaries. We are taught that being selfless makes us "good," "worthy," and "righteous," but we can't give from an empty cup. Joshua has found a way to help healers understand the importance of taking care of themselves so they can make an even greater impact on the lives of others.

Something I always appreciate about Joshua is that he is able to meet anyone for the first time and, within minutes, dive into the depths of their soul and profoundly understand their deepest needs. He quickly makes people feel seen, which catches them off guard and visibly captivates them. That is exactly what he has done with the healer community—he has been able to dive into the collective soul of healers, tune in to what they are needing, and deliver an effective solution in his distinctive Joshua style. He's tapped into a core theme that he, I, and so many other healers have struggled with.

With *Heal the Healer*, Joshua is paving the way, just like he did when he invented health coaching thirty years ago (now a billion-dollar industry), filling a gap in our broken medical system. He understands the unique challenges healers face and provides practical tools and strategies for overcoming these challenges. He does this while incorporating his mastery-level problem-solving skills and his way of breaking things down so they are easy for people to understand and integrate.

As someone who has been on the healing journey with Joshua for many years, I can attest to the transformative power of his teachings. Joshua's wisdom and guidance have helped me to heal my own emotional wounds and become a better healer. His teachings have also helped me to deepen my relationships with others, as I have learned to approach others with greater compassion and empathy.

What sets *Heal the Healer* apart from other books on the topic is Joshua's unique perspective on healing. He understands that healing is about more than fixing what is broken—it's about tapping into our innate power and potential. He believes that we are all capable of healing ourselves and others, and he empowers us to unlock this potential.

I am beyond thrilled that Joshua has brought this silent issue to the forefront and is helping healers all over the world reclaim their health, happiness, and ability to thrive while helping others. Whether you are a healer or simply someone looking to heal yourself, this book will provide the tools and guidance you need to embark on your own transformation.

ALEX ANZALONE

author, futurist, and Integrative Nutrition Health Coach

INTRODUCTION

♡

THIRTY YEARS AGO, I HAD A RADICAL IDEA to create a holistic nutrition school that would teach people that nutrition is about more than the food we put into our mouth. What we feed our hearts, minds, and souls is nutrition, too. This idea came after years of coaching others around nutrition, and noticing that talking about food was often just a gateway into discussing relationships, careers, spirituality, and other areas of people's lives that needed healing. I noticed there was a major gap in the healthcare system—a glaring lack of education and guidance around nutrition and emotional nourishment. This led me to pioneer the field of health coaching.

Health coaches take a holistic approach to wellness, considering all aspects of a person's life. They offer compassionate support through active listening, foster accountability, and guide others toward integrated well-being. Over the course of three decades, the Institute for Integrative Nutrition (IIN) has evolved into the world's largest nutrition school, empowering more than 150,000 students in 175 countries to transform their lives through diet and lifestyle and create meaningful careers as health coaches. In this time, I've observed thousands of IIN graduates on their journeys as health coaches. The demand for their services continues to rise as the healthcare system becomes more overwhelmed and more individuals seek to improve their physical, mental, and emotional well-being.

Something I've noticed from the earliest days of IIN is that almost all of the students attracted to the school exhibit a sort of "helper" persona. Like me, they are highly sensitive, perceptive people with a strong inclination to ease others' suffering and make a positive difference in the world. These characteristics make for natural healers, even before someone receives training in a healing profession.

But I know something now that I didn't know before. The very characteristics that make someone a good healer, like being highly sensitive, conscientious, empathetic, and intuitive, come with a downside; they make healers especially vulnerable to burnout, and can lead to a system imbalance that only worsens over time. We become better and better at helping others but often don't know how to get the help we need to heal ourselves.

As healers, we often struggle with recognizing our limits, setting boundaries, and asking for support. Instead, we go through our days striving to meet the needs of everyone around us. We can be like chameleons—shape-shifting to fill our roles in our families and society. These capacities make us especially good at caring for others but don't translate into self-care.

It's very common for people in helping roles and professions to experience burnout, compassion fatigue, and high levels of stress.[1] Some of us even develop physical ailments as a result of our ongoing quest to serve others. By the time things have progressed this far, we can be so disconnected from ourselves that we hardly notice. Many of us were never taught how to tune in to our feelings and care for our bodies. Instead, we keep pushing ourselves beyond our limits because functioning in overdrive is all we know. This constant self-neglect takes a great toll on us mentally, physically, emotionally, and spiritually.

Having dedicated my life to coaching, mentoring, and attentively engaging with healers both as a teacher and in my role as the director of IIN, I am keenly aware of the unique challenges healers face in today's world. I have witnessed firsthand what has worked for them and what has not, and I remain committed to helping them succeed.

WHY I WROTE THIS BOOK

After many years of working in overdrive, giving everything I could to IIN students and staff, I had a wake-up call when my health took a turn for the worse. I never imagined the IIN would grow to the size it has. I also never stopped feeling passionate about the school's mission, so I did everything I needed to do to carry it forward, even when that meant compromising my own health and happiness. There were times when I had to fight very hard to ensure the school would survive, to keep pushing the ball until I got it over the finish line. It was easy to devote all my time and energy to IIN when I had people from all over the world telling me I had changed their lives. I love helping people, so that feeling was kind of addictive. But my work-life balance was out of whack for too long. I burned out and paid the price for it. In 2018, I sold most of my interest in IIN to focus on my health. And I spent the last five years recovering and finding a healthy balance again.

During this period of time, we all experienced a state of emergency, which reached every corner of the globe and lasted for years. The coronavirus pandemic forced many of us to pause and reflect on what's important and what's not important in life. My mother passed away just before the pandemic, then my dad died of COVID-19 two years later. So, I had a lot to process in a short amount of time, and I learned a lot.

One thing I considered is how many healers spend their entire lives never slowing down, never taking the time to focus on their own healing. Many of us get absorbed in teaching, parenting, and caretaking or careers that involve helping others. These roles demand all our time and attention, distracting us from our own core wounds. I began to wonder: What is at the heart of a healer that makes us keep giving long after our batteries have run out? What is the driving force that makes us push ourselves beyond our means? For some of us, it's that we learned from a young age that we need to be selfless and good to be loved. For others, it's trauma we haven't totally worked through.

Often, we are subconsciously attempting to heal ourselves by healing others, but supporting others in their healing process is not a substitute for doing the work ourselves. This is why many healers lack self-confidence and experience imposter syndrome and feelings of self-doubt. We haven't dived into the depths of ourselves to figure out what keeps us up at night. We haven't received the level of support that we give so willingly to others.

In recent years, the world has seen an increase in burnout, anxiety, depression, loneliness, substance use, and suicidal thinking.[2] Even before the pandemic, millions suffered mentally, emotionally, and spiritually. Since then, things have only gotten worse, with more people overwhelmed by hopelessness, isolation, and grief and more reliant on prescription drugs.[3]

Meanwhile, healers face soaring demand and shrinking supply. According to one survey, around 100,000 nurses in the US left their jobs because of pandemic-related stress and burnout, and many more are expected to follow.[4] More than half of people in their forties are caring for both children and aging parents. With baby boomers aging into retirement and millennials starting to have babies—four million every year—care needs are ballooning at both ends of the generational spectrum. We need more care than ever before, yet we have less available, so we're reliant on overburdened working parents, family caregivers, and underpaid care workers overextending themselves.

Eager to move on from COVID, the world rushed back to business as usual—but there's an elephant in the room that needs to be acknowledged. We have collective PTSD, though very few people are talking about it. Just as many of us avoid processing early-life trauma, we put the pandemic behind us as quickly as possible. But unaddressed trauma doesn't go away. It lurks beneath the surface, continuing to have invisible effects.

With trauma at the root of some of the toughest issues the world is facing, the role of the healer has become more vital than ever. However, overburdened and undervalued healers cannot bear the weight of a broken system alone. Healers need healing, too, along with support.

This brings us to this book's core question: Who is

healing the healer? Many of us have no idea where to turn when we are the ones in need of help, and this is a major unaddressed issue in society today. For us to continue doing our work and make an even greater impact, we need to make a shift. We need to prioritize not only healing the public but healing the healer.

I wrote this book because I believe that with the right approach, healing the healer is possible. Trauma is often complex and deeply ingrained within the individual, so talk therapy is sometimes not enough on its own. To heal, we need to take an integrative, multi-pronged approach that focuses on healing through the mind as well as the body. Trauma-focused treatments and bodywork can help us process underlying emotions trapped in our bodies. This kind of work can be a great supplement to self-reflection, talk therapy, or counseling.

Additionally, we need to unlearn deeply ingrained patterns of thought and behavior that no longer serve us and develop the capacity to protect our energy. We all have a threshold when it comes to giving, and that's okay. You don't have to be completely selfless in order to be a good, caring person. In fact, when you don't show yourself compassion, it becomes impossible to consistently show compassion to others.

Most important, to heal, we need to connect with other healers who can support us in this process. Self-care is not a solo act. Maybe you have already figured out how to fill your life with things that nourish you: exercise, meditation, healthy food, and so on. That's all necessary. But we need to feel cared for by others in addition to caring for ourselves.

My mission is to support wellness workers and caregivers who feel emotionally exhausted, overworked, and overwhelmed and to inspire collective healing. As a supplement to this book, I am launching the Heal the Healer Live Experience to further the Heal the Healer movement and to bring healers together from around the world. More on this later.

WHO THIS BOOK IS FOR

If you feel drained from working in a helping profession or overcommitting yourself as a caretaker in your relationships and personal life, then this book is for you. In a world where institutional healthcare workers are increasingly overburdened, healers are asked to fill the ever-widening care gap, and that is a heavy lift. Whether you are a health coach, mental health professional, alternative medicine practitioner, parent, or caregiver, and whether your work is paid or unpaid, you understand the toll that caring work can take.

Although this book's primary audience is not healthcare workers such as doctors and nurses, my goal is to alleviate their burdens by addressing healer burnout holistically.

By empowering healers to enhance their self-care and caregiving abilities, I aim to bolster the healthcare system as a whole and promote a higher standard of health and well-being around the world.

HOW TO USE THIS BOOK

In Part I, we'll look at some common stressors healers face that can lead to burnout, such as emotional contagion, isolation, blurred work-life boundaries, and over-responsibility. I'll explain why common burnout solutions like productivity hacks and self-care often fall short and outline some obstacles that obstruct our path to healing.

In Part II, you'll learn how innate characteristics, childhood trauma, and social conditioning can set some people up to overfunction and neglect themselves, contributing to healer burnout later in life, and why certain personality types, like highly sensitive people, may be more prone to emotional exhaustion. You'll see why, in order to heal and prevent burnout, it's important to understand our formative influences, challenge ingrained assumptions, and live in greater alignment with our authentic selves.

In Part III, I'll walk you through setting boundaries as an essential part of protecting your energy and opening up space to experience more freedom and joy. We'll cover the importance of communicating your needs and setting limits with others, responding effectively when boundaries

are challenged, and establishing healthy limits for yourself. I'll explain why learning to say no without guilt and
prioritizing self-care requires self-awareness, self-trust,
and the courage to disappoint others when necessary.

Finally, in Part IV, you'll gain clarity on your authentic
values to guide your future actions. You'll evaluate your
current self-care resources, identifying the tools you are
lacking and the ones you would like to cultivate. And you'll
envision your ideal future, setting goals and planning your
next steps to getting there. This section is packed with tools
and strategies you can put into practice to transform your
life and break free from burnout, and ultimately emphasizes the importance of connecting with other healers.

This book is designed for you to work on yourself as you
journey through it. You'll find exercises where you can
assess your past and present and plan out your future.
Additionally, there are self-inquiry questions at the end of
each section. Please take time to reflect on these before
reading on. Even this self-inquiry process alone can contribute to your healing. To get the most from the process,
I recommend keeping a separate notebook where you can
jot down your answers. You can also work with an accountability partner, or simply close your eyes and meditate on
your answers.

To begin, grab a pencil or pen and take this initial self-
test. Circle your numbered response next to each statement.

HEALER BURNOUT SELF-TEST

	Strongly Disagree	Disagree	Neutral	Agree	Strongly Agree
I give more than I receive in most of my relationships.	0	1	2	3	4
I find it difficult to ask for help when I need it.	0	1	2	3	4
I have trouble communicating boundaries.	0	1	2	3	4
I feel guilty when I take time for myself.	0	1	2	3	4
I feel overwhelmed by my commitments and responsibilities.	0	1	2	3	4
I have difficulty concentrating.	0	1	2	3	4
I feel unappreciated and misunderstood.	0	1	2	3	4
I am highly sensitive.	0	1	2	3	4
I experienced trauma in my past that I have not healed from.	0	1	2	3	4
I have difficulty identifying my feelings.	0	1	2	3	4
I isolate myself from others when I am feeling low.	0	1	2	3	4
I am a perfectionist.	0	1	2	3	4
I have difficulty receiving compliments or gifts.	0	1	2	3	4
I experience chronic body pain, headaches, and/or I get sick often.	0	1	2	3	4
I ignore pain and symptoms in my body and put off going to the doctor.	0	1	2	3	4
I feel emotionally exhausted and numb.	0	1	2	3	4
I have a critical inner dialogue.	0	1	2	3	4
I feel lonely.	0	1	2	3	4
I feel undercompensated for the work I do.	0	1	2	3	4
I experience negative thoughts when I am not distracted.	0	1	2	3	4
I lack joy, play, and laughter in my life.	0	1	2	3	4
I make decisions according to what others need and expect from me.	0	1	2	3	4
I feel resentful when others don't acknowledge my efforts.	0	1	2	3	4

I have a strong need for approval from others.	0	1	2	3	4
I constantly worry about what other people think of me.	0	1	2	3	4
I say yes to unreasonable requests from others.	0	1	2	3	4
It affects me deeply when I witness other people's suffering.	0	1	2	3	4
I often feel impatient, anxious, and/or irritable.	0	1	2	3	4
I lack a sense of purpose unless I am helping others.	0	1	2	3	4
I avoid confrontation.	0	1	2	3	4
I experience sleep issues.	0	1	2	3	4
I have issues with food.	0	1	2	3	4
I am uncomfortable expressing my true feelings.	0	1	2	3	4
I rely on food, alcohol, or recreational/prescription drugs to help me relax.	0	1	2	3	4
I feel hopeless, helpless, and/or depressed.	0	1	2	3	4
I feel like if I don't keep pushing, everything in my life will fall apart.	0	1	2	3	4
I feel uncertain about what I want in the future.	0	1	2	3	4
I feel guilty when I assert myself.	0	1	2	3	4
I change myself to fit in with different people or groups.	0	1	2	3	4
I try to fix or rescue people.	0	1	2	3	4

Now, tally up your score by calculating the sum of your circled answers, and write down the total. Then use the following key to estimate your level of healer burnout.

0–40	Low or no healer burnout
41–80	Mild healer burnout
81–120	Moderate healer burnout
121–160	Severe healer burnout

PART I

WHAT'S BROKEN

CHAPTER 1
HEALER
BURNOUT

♡

IN PREPARING FOR THIS BOOK, I INTERVIEWED hundreds of self-identified healers from around the world, many of them IIN graduates, to gain insights into their healing journeys and struggles. Here are some excerpts from their stories:

"After becoming a health coach, I was ready to take on the world. I launched my website, podcast, and social media. I've been a listener all my life and was excited to have an audience to listen to me. But on my journey to heal others, I realized I needed healing, too. Raised in a first-generation Mexican household, I have been a caretaker for my family since I was very young. As a mom, I've always put my kids first, jumping up to tend to everyone else's needs before my own. I finally realized this came from the need to feel accepted and validated. This year, I decided to stop everything and finally prioritize my own healing so I can show up more authentically for my family."

—**WENDY** from Texas

"I'm dealing with burnout as the sole caregiver for my mom who has advanced Parkinson's. Being under constant stress and in a negative environment, I struggle to control my anger and frustration. I love my mother to death, but sometimes she drives me crazy. I understand how much she is suffering, but how much complaining can one endure? I feel lonely without any support from family, and it is not really possible for me to have a social life."

—**RICHIE** from Puerto Rico

"As a psychotherapist, I experienced burnout for the first time while working with cancer patients. I had a series of patients I identified with. Like me, they were divorced single moms of a similar demographic, and I found myself taking on their pain as if it were my own. I'd go home, cry, and have periods of fear that were overwhelming."

—**JONI** from Pennsylvania

"As a sandwich generation caregiver, I care for both my aging parents and a teen with mental health challenges. I am a healer out of necessity, not choice. The hardest thing about providing behind-the-scenes emotional labor is that it's not really acknowledged or valued by other family members, especially when weighed against what my partner does as the main breadwinner. I play therapist, teacher, mentor, and social worker—and I don't know anything about these professions, so I'm constantly improvising and trying to do all this self-training. When it comes to emotional labor, you can't point to it like you can point to other work, but it takes such a toll. I frequently battle exhaustion, frustration, and a sense of not doing a good enough job. I try to sneak in moments of self-care when I can, but it often feels frivolous given everything else I have to worry about in a day."

—**LYNNE** from Scotland

What these healers have in common is that they provide limitless amounts of care for others but lack care for themselves. Can you relate?

Dozens of other healers and care providers I interviewed shared that they are still recovering from pandemic-related stress and trauma. Many have faced grief over losing loved ones. Many care for aging parents or children with special needs. Many have struggled with their own health issues and/or disordered eating. Many have gone through major life transitions, such as divorce, career change, relocation, and empty nest syndrome. Many experienced a wake-up call like a health scare, accident, or mental breaking point, prompting them to slow down and prioritize their own well-being. Many struggle with upholding boundaries, protecting their energy, and letting go of perfectionism. Sadly, a few have even contemplated ending their lives at some point over the unmanageable burdens they carry.

While the work we do as healers can be extremely rewarding, without healthy boundaries, the pressure to "fix" people while absorbing their emotions can lead to deep psychological, even existential, exhaustion. Our strong passion to help others can drive us to overcommit, overextend, and overlook our personal needs. And our empathy can run low after a while when we fail to balance caring for others with caring for ourselves. I'll highlight more real-life healer experiences throughout the book as they relate to various topics.

WHO IS A HEALER?

When I talk about healing, I'm not suggesting anyone has the power to magically heal another person. Healers are the people who guide others in their healing process and set up the necessary conditions for healing to occur. That said, when I use the word *healer*, I refer to two groups of people in particular.

The first group is wellness workers. That includes alternative and holistic practitioners, health coaches, bodyworkers, Reiki practitioners, and everyone in between. It can also include therapists, social workers, and other mental health professionals. These are widely divergent occupations, but they all share some experiences in common; each involves working directly with people who are in need of healing or are working to improve their health and wellness.

I also use the term *healer* to refer to a particular personality type, one that predisposes people to alleviate others' suffering, regardless of their profession. Some people gravitate toward healing as caregivers, teachers, parents, and many other roles. Many of these natural healers are highly sensitive people with a giving nature. They tend to be conscientious, perceptive, intuitive, and empathic. They feel a heightened sense of responsibility for others, as they're often affected deeply by other people's suffering and pain. Many people in this category have told me they feel like old souls or misfits in society. Some have experienced adversity, trauma, and other life experiences that set them on a healing path. Others feel more like they were born with a spiritual calling to make the world a better place.

Healers in these two groups face plenty of the same challenges and are vulnerable to some of the same sources of stress. Often, healers actually fall into both categories.

STRESSORS HEALERS FACE

Helping others can be gratifying. Most of us feel fulfillment knowing we have made a positive impact on other people's lives. But caring can be stressful. It's easy to overlook the complexities that make healing work uniquely taxing. Let's explore some common challenges healers face.

First, healers take on a tremendous amount of responsibility for others. The health and well-being of those we care for may depend on the choices we make. And those choices hinge on how well we can assess our own skill level and ability to help in each case. Especially when starting out, healers often harbor insecurities about their ability to help. Even seasoned healers experience impostor syndrome from time to time. Then there is the opposite end of the spectrum: overconfidence. When a patient or client is worried or suffering, there's an expectation for healers to appear competent and reassuring. Play that role for long enough and you might convince yourself you're more skilled than you are. Whether it's insecurity or overconfidence at play, it can be hard to correctly assess your capabilities. And no matter how much expertise you have, you may still need to improvise to some extent, because every person you attend to and every circumstance you face is different. So, healing work requires balancing confidence and skill against humility and limitation.

Healers also have the jobs of helping people manage a wide range of emotions, like fear, anxiety, and shame, and managing their own emotional responses. Empathy is crucial for supporting others in their emotional processes. But with empathy comes vulnerability to emotional contagion and distress. It's hard to absorb other people's feelings without winding up feeling that way yourself. If you're highly sensitive, this effect is even stronger.

HEALER HIGHLIGHT

"As an empath, I absorb energy very easily, and I struggle with creating boundaries to protect myself. Whenever someone shares their pain or struggles—or whenever I see suffering in the world, especially involving innocents or animals—I carry that pain for days. I want to help solve all the problems in people's lives even if that means emptying my cup completely."—**SURYA** from Michigan

Another common occurrence is clients' situations triggering unresolved issues from your own past. For example, your client is struggling with grief over losing a parent, and it stirs up your grief over losing your dad. You may finish your workday and find you don't have the option of turning work off—you've got your own uncomfortable feelings to work through.

Another stressor healers face is difficulty getting clients or patients to cooperate in doing what they need to do to improve their condition. This might mean letting go of habits that are hard to break or deliberately choosing to face feelings they may desperately wish to avoid. Even when healers establish a foundation of trust and rapport with their clients, clients aren't always ready or willing to change.

Getting clients or patients to cooperate can be especially tricky when they have unrealistic expectations around how quickly they'll achieve results or how much effort will be required on their end. For example, health coaches often get approached by clients who are looking for a quick fix to losing weight. But coaches know real, lasting change comes from making gradual, sustainable lifestyle shifts. It's a journey that requires patience, commitment, and trust in the process. Some healers attract clients who are desperate because they've already tried everything else. Maybe you're their last hope, or they feel neglected by the healthcare system, which can make the stakes feel higher.

Adding to the list of challenges, healing work is not always clear-cut. Often when you're working to heal someone, you don't actually know the root cause of their health issue. A broken bone is pretty straightforward, but many conditions are more complex and mysterious. What if someone is dealing with infertility, a history of emotional neglect, or sudden allergies that seem to have come out of nowhere? Before you can help, you need to figure out what's actually causing their symptoms, and what, if anything, can be done about it. This may require troubleshooting and experimenting over a long period of time, advising interventions without knowing if they'll help, and managing patients' frustrations through the process of trial and error.

Because healing work can be so nuanced, it can be hard to tell when your job is over. How do you know when to let go? Similarly, how much responsibility can (or should) you take for another person's well-being? Although it's our job as healers to support and guide others, it is not our job to "fix" them. Ultimately, we need to understand that clients are experts in themselves. You have to work to earn someone's trust, then make sure they're not relying on you too much and ignoring their own instincts about what they most need.

Complete healing for your patient or client may not always be an option. To the extent you succeed at helping someone, you may receive praise and gratitude and feel pride in having made a difference. But given potential limits to how much you can help, you may instead be on the receiving end of their anger or disappointment. Could you have done more? Would someone else have done better? Maybe not, but it's hard to manage your own expectations about what can be healed and what can't. Sometimes, your role is to help someone accept a permanent change, loss of function, or chronic pain. That doesn't mean you've failed—but you may feel like you have anyway, and that can burden you with guilt. In some instances, if their issues fall outside your scope or you are unable to help them, you may need to make difficult decisions about referring clients to other professionals.

Lastly, being a healer can be lonely. Many are self-employed, so you're often making all these decisions on your own. You may not think of yourself as being isolated if you're interacting with clients all day. That's a lot of human contact. But it doesn't mean you're getting the assistance you need with the complicated judgment calls you're constantly having to make. Healers tend to work independently rather than as part of a team, and many work remotely, too. So, you don't get the social perks of a corporate setting—no "pizza Fridays" with coworkers. Instead, it's usually just you and the client, without much peer support or reassurance.

If you are a caregiver, you are likely dealing with a similar sense of loneliness and isolation, especially if you live in an environment where you do not have the necessary infrastructure, programs, and policies in place to support your caregiving responsibilities. You may feel as though your hard work and emotional labor set you apart from other people and go unnoticed.

There is a myriad of other challenges healers face, like being on call for patient emergencies, working odd hours, and liability concerns, to name a few. Given all this, it's not surprising that healers are especially susceptible to burnout.

THE COST OF CARING

Burnout is not unique to healers. Modern society encourages us to work too much, juggle too many tasks, and tolerate prolonged periods of stress and frustration. That's exhausting for anyone. Some aspects of burnout, however, are specific to healers. If you read over the list of stressors in the previous section, it's not hard to understand why. Healers spend a lot of time providing emotional support, witnessing pain and suffering, and taking on responsibility for other people's well-being. This takes an emotional toll on us and can lead to what's known as compassion fatigue: a state of exhaustion similar to burnout but uniquely associated with the stress of caregiving. Specifically, when care providers are unable to refuel and regenerate, their ability to empathize with others gradually lessens over time. If you start to feel numb or lose the ability to feel empathy, you may very well be tapped out emotionally. This is compassion fatigue.

There is also something called vicarious trauma, which refers to negative changes in a person's view of self, others, and the world, after empathically engaging with patients' trauma and suffering. For example, if you're a social worker who regularly counsels victims of domestic abuse, you might become more cynical, fearful, and withdrawn. Vicarious trauma is sort of like advanced compassion fatigue.

It is important to note that, compared to burnout, compassion fatigue and vicarious trauma are more complex forms of emotional distress, and may take longer to recover from. Depending on the kind of healing work you do and how vulnerable you are to emotional contagion, you might experience one or all three of these conditions.

For ease of reading, I will mostly stick to the terms burnout and healer burnout when referring to the state of stress and exhaustion healers experience. However, please keep in mind that compassion fatigue and vicarious trauma can be components of healer burnout.

Now let's take a look at the warning signs. Since overcommitted healers are often out of touch with their own bodies and tend to downplay their own needs, it can help to keep this list handy and refer to it as often as you need to.

Healer burnout may include the following:

- Difficulty coping with stress and/or feeling constantly overwhelmed
- Physical and emotional exhaustion
- Feeling empty or drained
- Impatience and irritability
- Difficulty concentrating
- Withdrawing or isolating from others
- Cynicism, pessimism, or negativity
- Loss of empathy or compassion
- Poor self-care (eating poorly, ignoring exercise, substance use)
- Sleep issues
- Feeling helpless, hopeless, or purposeless
- Decreased motivation and productivity
- Digestive issues, muscle tension, headaches
- Frequent panic attacks and/or constant anxiety
- Anger and resentment
- Memory problems
- Depression and/or existential despair

Nearly everyone experiences some of these symptoms now and then. They're part of being a human in the modern world. But healers work under unusually stressful conditions, making burnout prevention critical. Get to know your personal warning signs—how healer burnout manifests for you—so you can pace yourself and restore your strength, before it's too late.

Failing to address the signs of healer burnout means that unprocessed emotions and stress will continuously circulate through your body, gradually eroding your well-being over time. This leads us to the physical, mental, and spiritual costs of caring.

Chronic stress compromises nearly every bodily function—it raises blood pressure, lowers immunity, and disrupts digestion and hormones. Our sleep suffers and so does our nutrition, as we grab processed snacks to power through long days. Elevated cortisol also increases hunger, which can lead to overeating and interfere with absorption of nutrients. Chronic stress can even lead to reproductive problems and infertility, all because your body is in a prolonged state of fight-or-flight. For the body's systems to function properly, they need to receive the signal that they are safe. When this signal consistently doesn't come, the body is in a state of panic and disarray.

Healer burnout takes a toll on mental health, too. As a result of the emotional load they carry, healers often struggle with anxiety and depression. They may isolate themselves from others and give up on activities that used to bring them joy. They may lose their sense of purpose or feel helpless in the face of all the suffering in the world, which can also affect them spiritually.

COMPASSION IS A LIMITED RESOURCE

Personally, I have been known to push myself far beyond my means. One of my main mantras for as long as I can remember has been "We are all spiritual beings in a material world." When I consider my spirit, ageless and energetic, I feel limitless in my capacity to keep giving. It's like my soul doesn't recognize I'm inside a body, and I just want to continuously contribute to the lives of others. In my younger years, I could get away with it, but now that I'm older, it's a different story. Aging has forced me to slow down and pay closer attention to my body's cues and signals. My body lets me know when I have been oversharing my time, energy, and resources, and I do my very best now to listen.

Sometimes, we have enough time to do a thing but lack the necessary physical, mental, or emotional energy. Energy, like time, is a limited resource. We can only exert so much physical energy in a day before our bodies get fatigued. Similarly, we can only make so many thoughtful decisions in a day before our brains get fatigued. And we

can only exert so much caring energy before we become
emotionally exhausted. So, when we feel tired it could
mean a number of different things, depending on how we
have been spending our energy.

For example, if you spend your day at work responding to emails, it makes sense that by evening you would
feel too mentally exhausted to take on a project requiring
thinking and decision-making, so you may put off tasks
that require more brain power. If you spend your day
doing yard work or helping a friend move, you may not
have the physical energy to go to the gym afterward. And
if you spend your day caring for other people, you may feel
emotionally depleted by the end of it—too exhausted to
take on another person's emotions, even your own.

The fact that we have a limited supply of emotional
energy to spend taking care of others does not mean we
have a limited capacity for love or connection. But when
we continuously prioritize other people's needs, desires,
and comforts over our own, we are, in a sense, neglecting and abandoning ourselves; a neglected, abandoned
person cannot keep giving.

If you spend your days in a helping profession and your
evenings saddled with responsibilities for your partner,
kids, or others, you may be feeling emotionally numb or
overloaded. This does not make you a bad person. It's not a
sign that you are selfish or incapable of loving others. It is

instead a signal that you need some support, genuine con-nection, and a chance to rest your mind and nervous system. We need to feel cared for to keep providing care. We need to spend some of our caring energy budget on ourselves.

CHAPTER 2

BARRIERS TO SEEKING HELP

♡

HERE, I INVITE YOU TO DO A BRIEF EXERCISE with me to get more clarity about your intentions for the future. To start, contemplate your current experience of stress and burnout. Are there ways you're emotionally exhausted? Are there relationships in your work, or elsewhere in your life, that drain you? Are there changes you've been waiting or hoping to make but don't know how to achieve? You don't need to fill in all the details. Just tap into an overall sense of your current level of stress and burnout. It may help to write it down or speak it out loud: whatever you need to do to describe the problem in a way that is authentic to you.

Now, close your eyes and try to remember an earlier version of yourself—one who felt free. Maybe you felt a sense of freedom when you were a child or young adult that you haven't felt since. You weren't sacrificing yourself for others or trying to manage more than you were able to. Your life was more carefree in ways you might have taken for granted at the time. Recall what that freedom felt like. Maybe it wasn't a whole chapter of your life but a momentary flash. Whatever it was, connect with that feeling now.

It's possible you have never in your life experienced what it's like to live without feeling obligated to others or emotionally overwhelmed. In this case, try to connect with any image that represents freedom for you. Imagine someone else who represents this kind of balanced existence for you, or evoke a fantasy you have of what it could be like to feel freer.

See if you can contrast these two life experiences—the memory or fantasy you have of being free with your current state of stress and burnout. How different is the quality of life between the two?

Finally, consider what the future cost will be if your life remains as stressful as it is now. What are some possible consequences of continuing to operate in overdrive for another ten or twenty years? What will your health look like? What will your relationships look like?

One of the best ways to get motivated to fix a problem is to consider the cost of *not* fixing the problem. I see a lot of people put off thinking about the future because they are overwhelmed with the list of things they need to get done today. But it's kind of like ignoring squeaky brakes in your car. If you take your car to the mechanic right away, repairing your brakes might cost $200. On the other hand, if you keep putting it off, you'll eventually burn through the brake lining and the repair might cost $2,000 instead. Your body is your vehicle to get you through this life. If you ignore the warning signs of burnout and stress, you are likely to pay for it eventually. And by that point, the damage might be very hard to fix.

Hopefully, by now, you are seriously considering how healer burnout has been affecting your quality of life. Next comes the part where you lock in your intention—where you say, "I commit to treating this issue like the priority it is because my life depends on it!"

♡ *Where does solving the issue of healer burnout fall on your priority list?*

WHY A LOT OF BURNOUT SOLUTIONS DON'T WORK

Many of the resources that have been created to help people with burnout fall short for one reason or another. Some claim that the cure for burnout is finding ways to get more done in less time. You can find countless books and articles with titles like "Ten Tips to Get More Done in a Day." You can buy physical planners and organizers in every size, shape, and color. You can even find apps that help you organize your to-do lists and track your food, finances, and workouts. But is getting more done in less time the solution to burnout? Most people I know will just add more tasks to their schedule if they have more time, which will not help them feel better.

Some workplaces offer educational programs to counter employee burnout. However, people experiencing burnout aren't generally lacking education. More often, they lack support, connection, morale, and the opportunity to rest and restore themselves. By the time burnout has taken hold, they already feel stuck, exhausted, overworked, and powerless to change their situation. Plus, they don't have the time to attend another meeting or read a lengthy document. That only adds to their workload.

The self-care industry says the answer to everything is more meditation, more green juice, and more bubble baths. But the reality is that many healers are working around the clock earning a living and managing their caregiving responsibilities at home. All the self-care in the world isn't going to make their to-do list any shorter; it is essentially just another item to add.

While important and necessary, self-care has also become commodified by our culture, making it another source of stress, especially for those in financially limited situations. Self-care doesn't have to mean a membership to a pricey Pilates studio, or a Peloton, or a twelve-dollar smoothie from Whole Foods. Self-care can be as simple as taking a few deep breaths. It can be walking around your neighborhood or the nearest mall. But even when done right, there is only so much grounding and healing we can do on our own.

The reason these approaches to burnout don't work is because they aim to address the symptoms rather than the causes. Healing means addressing the sources behind the symptoms. It means asking questions like: Why are some of us more prone to burnout than others? Why do we have a difficult time recognizing our own limits or setting boundaries? Why is the feeling of responsibility for others such a weight to bear at times? All these questions can be answered by understanding the root causes of our burnout symptoms. For example, some of us have personality characteristics we were born with but have never learned how to embrace and account for. Some of us have deep-rooted emotional trauma that we store in our bodies. Many of us are conditioned by our upbringings or by society to comply with standards that don't make us happy or healthy. One of the hallmarks of healing is the extent to which we live in alignment with our authentic values, so this will be a step on our journey as well. Solving the burnout problem requires us to shift our ingrained behavior, which can be challenging in a fast-paced, grind-culture society. Once we learn how to set boundaries with our time, energy, and relationships, we'll be far more capable of nurturing ourselves in ways that make a true, lasting difference.

There's a second, equally important reason most burnout solutions don't work. All the hacks, education, and self-care in the world can't take the place of other people. At some point, we need to connect with and feel cared for by other human beings. No individual is meant to do it all alone, yet we have become more isolated than ever.

♡ *What burnout solutions have you tried so far? What has worked for you and what hasn't?*

REASONS WE DON'T SEEK HELP

It's hard to believe so many of us are lonely and isolated when we live on a planet with almost eight billion people. People are everywhere. There's no shortage. So, in theory, it shouldn't be hard for us to get the support we need, right? But we so often don't because there are obstacles that stand in the way, and we wear masks to hide unhealed trauma.

Read through the following list of reasons that we don't seek help to see if any of them may be obstructing your way toward healing. Which reasons resonate with you the most? Are there other reasons you don't seek help besides the ones on this list?

Superhero Syndrome

"I'm fine, really, I'm fine," is a good example of something you might hear a person with superhero syndrome say when they are, in fact, *not* fine. People with superhero syndrome believe their value comes from being needed, so they spend a lot of time and energy supporting others while minimizing their own needs. These individuals typically have a tendency toward enmeshment, people-pleasing, and codependency. They try to help, fix, or rescue others and take on more responsibilities than they can realistically handle. Superhero syndrome often goes hand in hand with perfectionism because people who take on the role of superheroes may have high standards for how things should be done. They may operate under the illusion that they're the only one who can help or do things right. They are also the last to admit they are hurt, and a person can't heal if they keep pretending nothing is wrong. Many healers struggle with this syndrome, which contributes to exhaustion and feeling overwhelmed.

Losing the Suffering Competition

Do you ever compare your suffering to other people's suffering, then invalidate yours because they seem to have it worse? For example, you might say to yourself, "Some people had abusive childhoods. Yeah, my father was overbearing, and my mother was distracted at times. But what gives me the right to get help working through my feelings about it?" Or you might think, "Lots of people don't have the opportunity to go to college, so I shouldn't complain about my student debt." It is dangerous to rank our suffering against other people's. Doing so puts us into a state of denial where we disallow ourselves from recognizing the pain of our own experience. We believe we're too privileged to be having a hard time. Unless we validate our own pain in whatever form it takes, we can't get the help we need to work through those feelings. And when we deny our own emotions, we tend to deny other people's emotions as well.

Toxic Positivity

Staying positive is a generally good idea, but enforcing positivity can be another form of denial. Toxic positivity involves dismissing negative or painful emotions and trying to maintain a happy, optimistic mindset at all times. An example of this would be a mother telling her son to "just be happy" while he is dealing with a painful divorce. The animated Disney Pixar movie *Inside Out* offers a beautiful illustration of how this can affect a child. In the film, young Riley's emotions spiral out of control after a move, illustrating how suppressing or neglecting certain emotions, like sadness, can lead to a lack of emotional resilience. Healthy emotional development requires acknowledging and embracing the full spectrum of emotions—not only

the positive ones. Unfortunately, the way many of us practice affirmations is part of the problem. In attempting to
improve our outlook or self-esteem, we tell ourselves things
we don't truly believe and pretend we're okay when we
aren't. We deny our real experience—or someone else's—to
avoid facing uncomfortable emotions.

False Resilience

Many healers are highly sensitive and possess an unmet
need to belong and be seen. For some of us, this comes
from not getting the love and nurturing we needed as
children or learning from a young age that we need to
suppress our needs for the sake of others. When we are
neglected as children, we learn to neglect ourselves. Later
on, as adults, we might seem resilient because we can tolerate not having our needs met, and it's what we are used
to. But is this true resilience? Or could it be an old survival strategy? Sometimes, what appears to be resilience is
actually armor we have developed to cope with not having
a secure attachment to our caretakers.

Being Overwhelmed

Life can sometimes feel like being in a car wash without
a car. There are all these things shooting at us from every
direction. So many people and things begging for attention. In American society, we live in a culture of excess. It

is nearly impossible to keep up with the constant influx of news, information, advertisements, and opinions that fill up our social media feeds and inboxes. Our consumer culture influences us to want more, buy more, have more. We have to make countless decisions each day about what to eat, what to wear, what to prioritize, and so on. Faced with this overabundance of choices and things to strive for daily, many healers feel overwhelmed and exhausted, which keeps them from taking action to improve their lives.

Isolation

Many of us are emotionally isolated. We may have friends on social media and, if we're lucky, a partner or a handful of friends we can rely on at a deeper level, but what's missing for most people is a supportive community. Society teaches us that we are strong if we are independent, but this is not necessarily true. We are strongest when we are authentically connected to other people. Countless people in the world right now are under the illusion that they are alone in their grief, suffering, or whatever they're experiencing. But the truth is that the majority of people out there are starving for connection and community.

Lack of Self-Trust

When we are forced from a young age to conform to various expectations set by our families, culture, and society, we learn not to trust our own needs and desires. We become disconnected from our bodies and our internal experiences. We ignore our intuitions. And we become lost. As a result, we may stay stuck in relationships, careers, or situations that aren't serving us. We may too easily trust other people, including authority figures, to know what's best for us rather than trusting our own experience.

The Comparison Trap

In the age of social media, we have constant access to other people's lives. Although much of what we see on social media is contrived in some way—photos are edited, and people post only the aspects of their lives they want others to see—we somehow still buy into the fantasy that it's all real. Then we compare ourselves to our friends, and even celebrities and strangers, and make up stories about why we aren't good enough. Of course, being stuck in loops of self-criticism and self-judgment causes major blockages in other areas of our lives. It's also exhausting. It takes a lot of energy to worry so much about how we look and how others perceive us. At the end of the day, it doesn't truly matter who has the most money, sex appeal, success, acclaim, or followers. Yet we give these things so much power in shaping how we feel about ourselves. Comparison is the thief of joy. We buy into the illusion that we are inferior based on narrow, curated depictions of other people's lives. Regardless of the parts of ourselves we put on display for others to see, we are all human. We all struggle with feelings of inadequacy, yet many people end up feeling alone in their suffering.

♡ *Which of these reasons for not seeking help resonate with you the most? Why? Are there other reasons you don't seek help besides the ones on this list?*

PART II

THE WOUNDED HEALER

CHAPTER 3

THE HEALER
PERSONALITY

♡

IF YOU'VE SPENT TIME WITH BABIES, YOU KNOW that each one is born with their own unique temperament. One baby is delighted by something new, loud, and flashy, while another finds that same level of stimulation overwhelming. Developmental psychologist Jerome Kagan discovered that easily overstimulated babies are far more likely to grow up to be introverts. He could predict, with impressive accuracy, whether a baby would be introverted or extroverted later in life. Despite this connection, Kagan also acknowledged that temperament is not destiny.[1] Humans are flexible creatures with the capacity for change. Starting out one way doesn't wholly determine what we might become decades later. However, understanding the differences in our innate dispositions helps us figure out how to manage our temperaments later in life.

Healers tend to be especially empathetic, perceptive, and sensitive. These traits allow us to attune to others and meet them where they are so that we can better help them get where they're going. But sometimes, these same characteristics get the better of us. We might be too sensitive or do a poor job maintaining a sense of separation between ourselves and the people we care for. This is how some of the same qualities that make us good healers also make us more susceptible to burnout. In this chapter, I'll explore some of the innate characteristics I've noticed in healers.

THE HIGHLY SENSITIVE PERSON

A good number of healers are highly sensitive people (HSPs) drawn to caring roles and healing professions, including health coaching. If you picked up this book, chances are you may know the term HSP already. And if you're anything like me, you may also have lived much of your life feeling alone in your experience of the world.

From the time I was young, I felt different from the people around me. There is a photo of me when I was five years old that illustrates this. In the photo, everyone around me is busy doing things, and I'm just sitting still and observing the scene, seemingly asking myself, "Where am I? How did I get here?" I was curious about the nature of reality even as a kid. So, I started questioning things around me. "What's really going on? Why are people behaving this way?"

Years later in adulthood, during one of my many trips to India, I was given a Sanskrit name. They called me Anand Nirav. *Anand* means joy, and *Nirav* means quiet or calm, like the kind of stillness you find at the center of a cyclone. I've always felt this to be a truthful description of how I feel. I am still on the inside, and there is all this swirling going on around me that I can't really relate to but which seems to be the consuming reality for most others. It feels as though I'm in neutral gear when everyone else is in drive.

For a long time, I didn't have words to describe why I felt like an outsider. I thought maybe there was something in my DNA that made me different—that I was programmed one way, and everyone else was programmed another way. I didn't cross paths with many people who shared my experience.

Then, in the 1990s, I came across the book *The Highly Sensitive Person* by Elaine Aron. According to Aron's research, HSPs have highly sensitive nervous systems.[2] We observe and feel things on a deeper level than most and pay attention to details in our environment that others might miss. It's like how when you ride a bicycle somewhere, you notice more than if you'd driven there in a car, and if you walk somewhere, you notice even more than if you'd ridden a bicycle. HSPs walk through life. We also have high empathy and a strong ability to tune in to other people's feelings.

Reading Aron's work, I thought, "Hallelujah! Finally, there is another person in the world who feels the way I do." I had spent my whole life up to that point searching for a term I didn't know existed. When I discovered the concept, an important puzzle piece fell into place.

Looking back now, I realize how isolating and alienating it was to be in the world for all those years with the sense that no one else was like me. Finding *The Highly Sensitive Person* was a revelation for me. It helped me realize I wasn't alone, understand myself better, and embrace my sensitivity as a strength, not a flaw.

When I started the Institute for Integrative Nutrition, I was surprised by how many of the students identified as highly sensitive people. I thought maybe 10 percent of students would relate to this term, but it was more like 70 percent. This was an astonishing realization. I went from being a total loner to thinking, "Oh my God, I've found my people." The highly sensitive students who were drawn to IIN had a specific way of thinking and learning. They were attracted to the school's curriculum and my style of teaching because it was creative, innovative, and participatory. I wanted to do more than lecture at students; I wanted to give them a chance to speak, to be heard and seen, and to create community.

As I learned from my own experience, as well as those of the students, being an HSP is both a blessing and a curse. It can be like having a sixth sense, a special antenna that picks up frequencies others can't hear. But with this heightened sensitivity comes a greater responsibility to care for ourselves. Because we absorb other people's energy and emotions, we often need a lot of alone time to rest our senses and recharge. We are also very sensitive to our environments. For example, I feel overstimulated when I spend a lot of time in big cities filled with constant noise and commotion. I do better in environments that are tranquil and calm, which is why I live in a small town in the woods.

Because HSPs are extra sensitive to their surroundings, everything becomes magnified. This is one reason we may experience burnout more quickly and more intensely than others. It's the way we are wired, but it doesn't mean there is something wrong with us. It just means we need to be mindful about how we manage our energy, including who we share it with and what kinds of environments we put ourselves in.

If you're a highly sensitive person, you were also a highly sensitive child. Highly sensitive children are influenced more by their emotional and physical environments than other children. They are more easily overwhelmed by high levels of stimulation, sudden changes, and the emotional distress of others.[3] They are also more likely to feel painfully disconnected from self-involved or emotionally distant caretakers and to internalize the pain they experience. In the next chapter, I talk about the kinds of developmental traumas some of us endured growing up. For highly sensitive kids, the effects of those experiences are often amplified.

Something else to note is that sensitivity is valued differently in different cultures. Western society tends to reward thick-skinned people who are less sensitive. If you are highly sensitive and living in the United States, you may feel pressure to mimic less-sensitive people to fit in. Maybe you have pushed yourself to go to concerts, sporting events, and loud parties. Or maybe you've tried saying yes to going out more than one or two nights a week but felt exhausted and irritable afterward.

Sadly, living in a culture where sensitivity is not understood or encouraged can lead to low self-esteem and a lack of self-trust in people who are more sensitive. Many HSPs are told to toughen up from a young age, which denies our natural tendencies and makes us feel shame. We might also be misperceived as shy or unsociable when we are just temporarily overstimulated.

To help you determine whether you might be an HSP, I recommend taking the self-test available at hsperson.com.

Additionally, the aspects of high sensitivity are summarized here using the acronym DOES: depth of processing; overstimulation; emotional responsivity/empathy; and sensitivity to subtleties. To learn more, visit hsperson.com/faq/evidence-for-does/.

♡ *Are you highly sensitive? If so, does it feel like a blessing or a curse? Regardless of whether you identify as a highly sensitive person or not, have you found ways to stay open and empathetic without getting overwhelmed and caught up in other people's feelings?*

THE CHAMELEON QUALITY

Many healers are people-pleasers. They are able to go with the flow and tend to have a chameleon quality. They shapeshift to fit into an unusually wide range of environments. If this is you, you might put on a certain mask at work so your boss sees you as hardworking and reliable. Then you come home and put on a different mask for your family, always being patient and in control around your kids. And when the weekend rolls around and you socialize with friends, maybe you put on yet another mask so people perceive you as fun, interesting, and sociable.

It's true that it can feel like a superpower to be able to transform into whatever other people want you to be. But on the downside of this chameleon power, most healers I know have a hard time taking up space and saying, "This is who I am. Deal with it." This is a problem because that's what the rest of the world does seemingly without issue, which puts people-pleasers at a disadvantage.

Over time, I have seen chameleon-like healers compromise to the point of convincing themselves that their lives are okay when they are noticeably unhappy. It's like the popular meme taken from K.C. Green's webcomic "On Fire," in which a cartoon dog sits in a room engulfed in flames and simply says, "This is fine." When healers fail to take ownership of their own lives, they end up as supporting actors to other people's leading roles. For example, let's say you dream of living near the ocean in Florida, but your partner wants to stay in Minnesota. If you're a chameleon adapting to everything, you might say, "Well, it isn't *that* bad. The place we live isn't *that* cold."

Healers are usually conditioned to be helpful and cooperative. They are taught that giving makes them good people. Sometimes a religious upbringing keeps us tethered to the idea that we are selfish if we fail to serve the people around us. We conform to these ideas to fit in. But shapeshifting and self-sacrificing for the sake of pleasing others leads to self-denial, resentment, and compounding stress. Hiding and denying your authentic self is not true strength, even though it requires a huge amount of work and effort.

♡ *How much do you shapeshift to fit in with your*

environment? Is the way you present yourself mostly stable, or does it change a lot depending on who you are around? Do you ever find yourself being too agreeable?

INTUITIVE VERSUS SENSING TYPES

The Myers-Briggs Type Indicator is probably the most widely used personality assessment tool. The test measures a range of psychological and behavioral preferences and categorizes people into types based on how they perceive information and make decisions. For example, you'll learn by taking the test whether you are an intuitive type or a sensing type. Intuitive types focus on the big picture—they pay attention to overall impressions, feelings, and meanings embedded in the information they receive. Sensing types, on the other hand, pay more attention to concrete facts and details. They tend to focus more on what is actual, present, current, practical, and real.[4]

For most of the Myers-Briggs personality characteristics, the population tends to be evenly divided between the two sides. The one exception seems to be intuitive versus sensing; at least two-thirds of the people who take these tests fall on the sensing side of the spectrum.[5] When it comes to healers, however, it's the opposite. The majority of healers seem to be intuitives. This quality is great for seeing deeply into complex situations, reading between the lines, and coming up with creative responses. These are real advantages. However, as a healer, you may be less skilled when it comes to figuring out practical steps for helping others or managing your own needs. You might feel overwhelmed by the nitty gritty details of managing your own resources or running your business, which can contribute to healer burnout.

Intuitive types could often benefit from strengthening their sensing skills to stay grounded, care for themselves. and keep their work sustainable. It's the oxygen mask principle: you can't continue contributing to others unless you first make sure your own needs are met.

If you want to test yourself, I recommend the website 16personalities.com. They offer their own modified version of the Myers-Briggs test that is user-friendly, insightful, and free. Or you can visit myersbriggs.org for more information.

♥ *Where do you fall on the spectrum of intuition and sensing? What are your related strengths? What related weaknesses might you need to learn to compensate for?*

PERFECTIONISM

Do you hold yourself to very high standards? Do you kick yourself after you do something less than perfectly? Do you feel like you need to do everything without help? I am not personally a perfectionist, but I know many healers who are. High standards, critical thinking, and self-determination are all valuable resources to have—so long as you're able to be open and flexible when you need to. The problem with perfectionism is that it is often guided by stubbornness, inflexibility, and a lack of self-compassion.

Because perfectionists are concerned with others seeing them as self-sufficient, they often avoid asking for help when they need it. They also tend toward self-criticism, which can lead to increased stress, loneliness, and burnout. Being self-critical usually means being more critical of others, too. At the root of perfectionism, you will often find feelings of inadequacy or shame. Most perfectionists believe they need to prove their worth through their accomplishments and how they appear to others. Without external achievements, they feel as though they lack intrinsic value. Perfectionists may not realize how much this tendency prevents them from building true intimacy in relationships. Real intimacy requires allowing others to witness your vulnerability and pain.

People sometimes ask me how I've managed to be successful without being a perfectionist. You've probably heard the saying, "Done is better than perfect." I've taken it to heart. Trusting the process and allowing things to be *good enough* means not much stands in the way of me continuing to try new things, including in my work.

Take writing this book, for instance. I could, no doubt,

have spent years revising, improving, and polishing it to perfection. But if I'd done that, you wouldn't be reading it now! I wanted to put it out into the world quickly to start making a difference. That choice also means I'll get feedback sooner rather than later about how useful it is to readers. I can then use that feedback to make a later edition of the book far better than if I was still thinking it through all on my own.

I ran IIN with this same philosophy in mind. The school changed dramatically over time, never perfect but always evolving. In general, I think offering something is better than offering nothing. If perfectionism prevents you from trying something new, remember this: something can be improved on later, but nothing can't!

♥ *Does perfectionism stop you from enjoying the things you're good at? Does it stop you from trying new things?*

You may or may not relate to the characteristics discussed in this chapter. There are many helpful personality typing systems and countless potential categories to divide people into. While no individual can be defined by a single label or personality test, having self-knowledge about how we process information and relate to others empowers us to take better care of ourselves. With self-knowledge, we develop greater awareness of the unique traits that set us apart from other people and can better attune to our unique needs. For example, if you are highly sensitive, you might need more time to recover from highly stimulating experiences—and that's okay. If you ignore your differences and try to conform to the way other people operate, you will potentially suffer from more exhaustion and pain. The fact that you need to take care of yourself in specific ways as a healer doesn't make you weak.

CHAPTER 4

WHAT NEEDS TO BE HEALED

♡

HAVE YOU HEARD THE TERM WOUNDED HEALER? Carl Jung originated the idea of the wounded healer to describe caregivers who feel compelled to help others because they themselves are wounded. He suggested that people are often drawn to healing professions like counseling, psychotherapy, nursing, etc., because they are subconsciously seeking to heal their own pain.[1]

By drawing on their own experiences of suffering, trauma, and/or illness, wounded healers deeply empathize with those they help. Their pain informs their approach and draws them to alleviate others' suffering. However, wounded healers need to be careful to not overidentify with clients or patients or unconsciously project their own healing needs.

I bring up the wounded healer to provide another lens for exploring what makes a healer. In the previous chapter, we looked at innate temperaments and characteristics: the nature side of things. Now, we're going to examine the nurture side. What early life experiences lead to self-sacrifice and an exaggerated sense of responsibility for others? Some formative experiences, particularly childhood trauma or neglect, are common to wounded healers and later contribute to healer burnout.

I think a lot of healers (including, at an earlier stage in my life, myself) would say, "Trauma? I don't have any trauma." We're so good at dismissing trauma when it comes to ourselves, yet our behaviors reveal otherwise. I've seen healers try to eat perfectly, exercise perfectly, and develop perfect routines to convince themselves they are in control of their lives. Others overextend themselves helping others, leaving no time for self-care. When we look behind the curtain, these behaviors are often compensating for old feelings of powerlessness and lack of control. We try to be perfect to fulfill an underlying need for validation and acceptance. We focus on others' problems to avoid facing our own unresolved issues.

Although many healers appear super high-functioning, we are not always thriving. A lot of us grew up in situations where we lacked nurturing. As a result, we may never have learned to nurture ourselves. Until we acknowledge and address our childhood wounds, we can't recognize how many of our behaviors we adopted as survival mechanisms. By examining the wounded healer, we can better understand the roots of common healer tendencies. This awareness empowers us to heal these wounds and prevent burnout.

EARLY CONDITIONING

During our formative years, we take in information from our environments at a rapid rate. Some people think babies and infants don't absorb much because they don't understand language, but the opposite is true. The younger we are, the more malleable our brains are. Before children can speak, they are highly attuned to nonverbal forms of communication. They pick up on tension, despair, and hostility in the people around them. Our earliest life experiences have the greatest impact on our brain development and functioning.

From the time we are born, we rely on our caretakers to help us interpret the world around us. Their sensibilities and worldviews shape our sense of self-worth, our earliest and most fundamental beliefs, and the kinds of relationships we choose throughout our lives.

If you work in a healing profession, especially as a health coach or mental health professional, you've probably encountered what I call the magic of mirroring.

Something comes up for one of your clients or patients, and you realize, "Whoa! The same issue is coming up in my life!" Miraculously, our clients tend to mirror the exact things we need to work on. When this happens, it's an opportunity to learn about what we need to heal in ourselves. Healing ourselves makes us better able to heal our clients without getting triggered in the future.

HEALER HIGHLIGHT

"As the owner and founder of the Center for Nutritional Healing, I've worked as a healer since 2014. I am naturally inclined to help others and a natural born teacher. When I was a teenager, my parents' marriage was unraveling, and I truly believed I could save it. My mother told me, "You're just the daughter," but I continued with every ounce of me trying to fix it anyway. This is my nature and how I tend to be with every person that walks in my office door."

—CINDY from Pennsylvania

DEVELOPMENTAL TRAUMA

Now, let's take a look at trauma, which so many healers experience during childhood and adolescence. When most of us think of trauma, we think about experiences such as violent assaults, serious accidents, the sudden loss of a loved one, and natural disasters. Trauma is defined as the lasting emotional response that results from living through a distressing event.[2] But lasting emotional responses don't always stem from single, acute, or life-threatening experiences. Developmental trauma, also known as complex trauma, involves multiple traumatic experiences that are chronic or prolonged over a period of early development. This can take the form of ongoing neglect, bullying, or abuse, but it also comes from exposure to other sources of stress in one's home. These range from obvious stressors, like witnessing domestic violence, to more subtle or ambiguous stressors, like a parent withholding love only some of the time. These repeated stressors have cumulative effects, some of which are even more impactful than a single traumatic episode. To get a better sense of your early stressors, let's take a look at the four parenting styles, commonly recognized by psychologists, that shape our personalities and coping mechanisms: the *authoritative* parenting style, the *authoritarian* parenting style, the *permissive* parenting style, and the *neglectful* parenting style. Each of these parenting styles has a different effect on a child's development. While authoritative parenting is closest to the ideal, authoritarian, permissive, and neglectful parenting styles can influence children to overfunction, deny their own needs, or struggle in relationships later in life.

It's important to mention upfront that a child's experiences are shaped by the interaction between their temperament and their environment. Two siblings raised by the same parents can have two very different experiences of their family. If one sibling is highly sensitive, they might experience developmental trauma as the result of ongoing parental neglect or perceived neglect, while the other less sensitive sibling might not perceive neglect at all. Also, parents rarely fit neatly into one of these categories. Typically, they fit into more than one category or shift between them at different times.

Authoritative Parents

Authoritative parents are warm, responsive, and supportive. They set realistic expectations and boundaries for their kids and establish the structure young people need to thrive while allowing their kids freedom and independence. These are the parents who take time to have open discussions with their children. If they set a rule or boundary, they'll explain why they are putting the rule or boundary in place so that their kids develop trust and understanding. They encourage their children, believe in them, and push them to grow. Children of authoritative parents are typically happy, active, sociable, and have high self-esteem.

Authoritarian Parents

These are the parents who love the phrase, "Because I said so." They give their kids rules for how they should behave, but these rules are often detached from reason, explanation, and compassion. As a result, children of authoritarian parents learn to suppress their instincts and spontaneous impulses. They often organize themselves around whatever they're expected to do to avoid getting in trouble. Later in life, they might find themselves in submissive roles in relationships because they are used to following rules without asking questions. Or they may do the opposite by stepping into a dominant role once they have the chance, as that's what's been modeled for them. Either way, they might come to see relationships as power struggles or zero-sum games. They may not know that genuinely collaborative relationships are possible—or even be able to recognize one if it comes along!

♥ *Did your caregivers help you to understand why rules mattered by enlisting your cooperation in creating a healthy family environment? Or did they dominate you with rules for rules' sake and punish you if you did not obey them? If the latter, are there relationships in your life currently that are characterized by one person exerting power over the other?*

Permissive Parents

If your parents or caregivers were permissive types, you probably enjoyed the freedoms that make childhood fun but lacked the structure young people need to thrive. You may never have learned how to recognize your own limits, set boundaries, curb impulses, delay gratification, or endure the challenge of doing things that are hard. In short, your childhood lacked discipline. People who grow up in these conditions often have a hard time maintaining structure later in life. They can be indecisive, noncommittal in relationships, and lack an inner sense of stability. They may not be as capable as others raised in stricter environments that mirror the institutional structures of society.

♡ *Growing up, did you learn how to work within limitations, make choices, and tolerate discomfort? Or were you given freedom without ever learning how to manage it? If the latter, have you since been able to develop discipline and a strong sense of self?*

Uninvolved/Neglectful Parenting

The uninvolved parenting style, sometimes called the neglectful parenting style, refers to caregivers who take a hands-off approach with their children. For the most part, these parents allow their kids to do what they want. This could either be by choice or by circumstance, as uninvolved parents are often absent physically, mentally, or emotionally. Children who grow up with uninvolved parents receive the message over and over again that their needs are not important. As a result, they may struggle with low self-worth, anxiety, depression, or other mental health and/or behavioral issues.

♡ *Were you raised by caregivers who took an active role in your welfare and set limits to keep you safe? Or did they neglect your needs and leave you to figure things out for yourself? If the latter, have you figured out ways to set limits for yourself as an adult and surround yourself with support?*

Now that we've taken a look at the four parenting styles, I want to mention a few additional childhood experiences that may contribute to the psychology of the wounded healer. See if you identify with any of the following.

Parentification

Parentification, I have noticed, is especially common among healers, and sets them up to be caretakers throughout their lives. Parentification involves a role reversal between parent and child, in which the child acts as the parent and the parent acts more like a child.[3] Parentified children become caretakers from an early age—for themselves, parents, and often siblings as well. For example, they might take responsibility for practical household tasks like cooking, cleaning, and paying bills. They might also put their younger siblings to bed and help them with their homework.[4] Parentification also occurs when parents rely on their children for emotional support, expecting their kids to carry their heavy burdens and solve their adult problems. For example, Carlos grew up with an alcoholic mother and an absent father. As a kid, it was not uncommon for Carlos to find his mom passed out on the couch from drinking too much. Whenever this happened, Carlos would take off his mother's shoes, cover her with a blanket, and place a glass of water on the table beside her. Other times, Carlos's mother would complain to him about how lonely she felt as a single parent, relying on Carlos for emotional support. Parentification is more common in families where a parent struggles with addiction or mental illness. But it can happen in any family where parents lack emotional maturity, stability, and a sense of responsibility. As a result of growing up without attentive and loving parents to offer encouragement, guidance, comfort, and validation, parentified children often feel alone, overwhelmed, scared, and angry. As adults, they may have a hard time connecting with their emotional needs and trusting others. They may also continue to be overly responsible in their adult relationships, tending toward compulsive caretaking and attracting individuals in need of rescuing or fixing.[4]

♥ *Did you get to enjoy the carefree experience of childhood? Or did you miss out on childhood because you were expected to play the role of an adult for as long as you can remember? If the latter, how does that affect the way you live your life now?*

Lack of Attunement

A lot of healers grow up with parents who are well-intentioned but lack the self-awareness or emotional skills to attune to their children's emotional needs. I often hear people say, "My parents were good parents. They gave me everything I needed—food, shelter, a college education." It is possible to be well taken care of materially and still grow up feeling emotionally alone. If your primary care-takers were self-involved, you may have learned to put their needs before your own or work unreasonably hard to get their attention. If they were available but lacked emotional intelligence, they may have given you plenty of attention of the wrong kind or at the wrong times, like being overly critical, demanding, or imposing on your privacy. When a caretaker is consistently there for you, aware of your needs, and doing their best to meet them, several important things happen: you internalize a sense of security, the basis of secure attachment later in life; you develop a healthy model of what intimacy is; and because you have some-one paying enough attention to your particular needs, you learn to identify those needs. On the other hand, if there's no one around who attunes to you, or if that attunement is unreliable, the opposite occurs: you internalize a sense of insecurity; you don't learn much about how to create inti-macy in relationships; and because your feelings are not seen and validated by others, you learn not to trust your-self. Attunement is something certain people never think about, but it's crucial to our emotional development. Its presence establishes a foundation for healthy relationships, while its absence can leave us on shaky emotional ground, especially if we are sensitive and highly attuned ourselves.

♡ *When you were young, did your caregivers tune in to your emotional needs and provide a consistent source of love? Or were they unable to recognize or meet your emotional needs? In either case, how has that influenced your sense of self and your style of relating to others?*

Impossible Expectations

Children raised by parents who hold them to very high standards feel they must continuously prove they are worthy of love. Parents like this keep raising the bar so that the child is in a constant state of earning. For example, a high-expectation parent might punish a child for getting below a B on a test at school. Or they might push their child unreasonably hard at sports, rewarding them when they do well and ignoring them when they do poorly. As a result, children of parents with impossibly high expectations learn that love and approval are conditional, based on what they achieve. They often become people-pleasers, perfectionists, and overachievers. They work to earn attention, affection, and validation from the people around them, often at the expense of their own happiness.

♡ *Growing up, were you given support to learn and grow*

with realistic expectations? Or were you constantly made to feel like you were never good enough? If the latter, have you found a way to detach your sense of worth from your sense of accomplishment?

Walking on Eggshells

When one or more of your caregivers are emotionally fragile, volatile, or violent, you learn to maintain vigilance for signs that something might blow up. You're always walking on eggshells, managing your own behavior in the hope of managing your caregiver's unstable emotions. In this sort of environment, you wind up focusing all your attention on keeping yourself safe from the people who are supposed to protect you. Because we're so adaptive when we're young, a consistent, underlying feeling of danger or dread can start to feel normal. We get so used to feeling that way, we don't realize that life can be different. Children in these environments often grow into adults who are hypervigilant and hyperattuned to other people's moods, feelings, and needs. As adults, they may do a lot of emotional work in relationships to try to help or change people who don't want to change themselves.

♡ *Were you raised in an atmosphere of safety by caregivers who took responsibility for their own emotional states? Or did you need to develop some kind of vigilance to manage the emotions of the people around you?*

If the latter, are there ways you continue to do that now?

Violence and Abuse

People whose childhoods include violence or abuse may grow into adults who feel defenseless. They are likely to have an especially difficult time with boundaries because they were forced into situations they couldn't say no to. They may also have trouble speaking up for themselves, trusting themselves, and detecting when they are being taken advantage of. Kids who never felt safe often become adults who don't know how to establish safe environments for themselves or create safety for the people around them.

♡ *When you were growing up, did your caregivers keep you safe from harm? Or did you endure abuse, violence, or disempowerment? If the latter, have you since been able to reclaim a sense of your own power?*

Cumulative Effects

Do any of these patterns reflect what you experienced as a child? Of course, there are other kinds of upbringings not mentioned here. But this is how developmental trauma can form as a result of ongoing experiences of trauma and neglect. Our early attachments have a huge impact on the attachments we form later in life. They become the blueprint for all our relationships. So, to move forward into healing, it is important to bring attention to the roles we learned to play when we were younger. From there, we can examine our present-day relationships and determine to what extent we are still playing those roles and whether they're serving us.

♡ *If you could go back in time and ask your child self what they most want and need, what would your child self say? In what ways has your relationship with your parents or caregivers affected your adult relationships?'*

A Note for Parents

If you are reading this chapter as a healer who is also a parent yourself, or perhaps one of the sandwich generation (those caring for children and parents at the same time), you might be thinking, "Oh no! There are so many ways to mess up my kids! How can I possibly get everything right?" It's a valid question, especially if you didn't have particularly healthy examples of parenting when you were growing up. We need a license to drive a car but not to do the much more complex job of raising children. Parents aren't given a manual on how to parent.

That said, I want to invite you to take a big breath with me and momentarily release all those concerns. The fact that you're even curious about how to best nurture your child's development shows that you're already living in a far more enlightened paradigm than almost every parent as recently as a couple of generations ago. Perfect parenting isn't possible nor necessary. The very act of bringing awareness to the question of how to parent well already gets you halfway there. Remember that this is a book about burnout and healing, not about putting more pressure on yourself than you already do. So, I invite you to trust that if you take care of your own healing, your children will reap the benefits—without you needing to become a super parent.

♡ *Do you still carry imprints of less-than-ideal parenting from your childhood? Are there things you never learned about parenting from your caregivers? What do you most wish to heal in yourself to create the kind of family you wish you could have grown up with?*

GENERATIONAL TRAUMA

According to clinical psychologist Dr. Joy DeGruy, generational trauma refers to the cumulative emotional wounds inflicted on a group of people over generations stemming from massive historical trauma.[5] In her book *Post Traumatic Slave Syndrome*, DeGruy examines the impacts of slavery, systemic racism, and oppression on present-day African Americans.

DeGruy explains that the brutal traumas inflicted during slavery caused untreated post-traumatic stress for those enslaved, affecting their ability to cope and heal from the violence. These trauma responses and coping mechanisms were then passed down to subsequent generations through genetic changes, parenting practices that unconsciously perpetuate trauma, and ongoing oppression and discrimination that retriggers trauma. This contributed to instability in African American families, including higher rates of violence, substance abuse, and strained relationships, continuing to impact descendants today.

Whether or not we know what our parents and ancestors went through—in fact, even if we are raised apart from our biological families—their trauma can affect us epigenetically. This means we can absorb our forebearers' beliefs formed during tough times or periods of violence as well as the strategies they developed for surviving hardship and we can epigenetically inherit the pain and stress they carried.

Both of my parents were Holocaust survivors. When I was growing up, they would tell me horrific stories about how often they escaped death "by the skin of their teeth." One time, when my mother was fourteen, she was forced into a gas chamber at Auschwitz, but for some reason the gas didn't work that day, and she miraculously survived. Another time, she snuck out of line to get some much-needed water with her friend, when the guards started shooting at them. They jumped into the cistern to escape, and when my mother opened her eyes, the water was red. Her friend was dead, but she was spared. She was just sixteen years old.

For the most part, my father didn't talk about the war. He said the things he experienced were too awful to share. But he once told me about the death march at the end of the war. As Allied troops approached the German front lines, my father, along with thousands of other prisoners, were forced to evacuate the camp and walk for days. These marches came to be called death marches because so many died along the way. Prisoners suffered from cold and starvation. They had no winter clothing—many didn't even have shoes. If anyone trailed behind because they grew too tired or weak, the soldiers shot them dead so they wouldn't slow down the group.

"Conditions were so deplorable," my father said, "that when someone died, others would scramble to take the coat or shoes off the dead body. We lost our humanity trying to survive." After marching for days, my father grew weak and sick, so his brother carried him on his shoulders. My father lost consciousness after that. The next thing he remembered was waking up in a hospital, and the war was over. But he was never able to find his brother. Nor was he able to come to terms with the fact that his brother might have died saving his life. Thirty years later, he was still placing ads in Jewish newspapers around the world, trying to find him.

Because my parents survived so much when their

WHAT NEEDS TO BE HEALED

families and so many others did not, they experienced what is referred to as survivor's guilt. This is part of the reason they devoted so much of their lives to helping others. For many years, my father worked for a nonprofit assisting people with immigration issues, and my mother loved volunteering to help people in need. They made frequent charitable contributions and were exceedingly generous with friends and family.

The unspeakable trauma my parents went through shaped the kind of people they were and the kind of person I became. For example, I have always been great at avoiding confrontation. There's a part of me that will say, "Okay, I'm at peace with that," even as I work to contain my resentment. Eventually, I figured out that I had learned to do this as a child. Because my parents had suffered so much, I tried not to add to their pain by complaining. I also felt that I didn't have the right to complain or have problems, because anything I could be going through was insignificant compared to what they had endured. So I suppressed my feelings and needs to avoid upsetting my parents. This became a problem later in life as I resisted sharing my true emotions in relationships because I didn't want to be a burden to others. What started for me as an adaptive behavior in childhood—a survival strategy developed to avoid conflict—became maladaptive later in my life.

Ultimately, generational trauma touches everyone. Your

parents may not have grown up in a war-torn country, but you don't have to go back many generations to find wars, slavery, persecution, deprivation, upheaval, or displacement in any country's history. Generational trauma permeates entire cultures, becoming embedded in structures of family life, religion, education, recreation, and commerce. It shapes worldviews in subtle yet profound ways. Considering how prior generations' beliefs and trauma responses shaped our current culture helps us understand the roots of ongoing suffering as well as resilience.

Healers may feel especially impacted by generational trauma, and compelled to help others because of the emotional burdens they carry. This makes it critical for healers to confront rather than avoid their trauma, or the cycle continues. Healing generational trauma requires processing painful emotions and memories, rebuilding self-worth, and creating healthier coping habits over time.

♥ *Consider what you know about your parents or caregivers. What traumas did they experience that you are aware of? What traumas did they never talk about? Do you think their trauma was mostly processed or unprocessed? How about your grandparents and great-grandparents?*

CHAPTER 5

THE SOCIAL
FORCES THAT
SHAPE US

♡

FROM THE FOOD WE EAT AND THE CLOTHES
we wear to how we behave and what we desire, our
social conditioning influences every domain of our lives,
instilling in us countless norms, rules, and conventions
that govern how we live. It is a powerful, invisible force
that we are constantly engaging with. As healers, challenging the social expectations and limiting beliefs we have
internalized may feel destabilizing, but it is an essential
part of preventing burnout and living more authentically.
Examining our conditioning allows us to identify which
inherited beliefs and behaviors serve our highest good,

and which we need to release so we can follow our soul's purpose. Liberating ourselves from the confines of the past is healing. It lets us get out of our minds and return to the wisdom of our original selves. In this chapter, we'll look at a few ways our conditioning influences us and how questioning what we've been taught can set us free.

Conditioning happens in two ways. First, our behavior is shaped when we're rewarded for certain behaviors and punished for others, especially during childhood. Societies train young people to become members of that society by making them feel good when they do what they're *supposed to* and bad when they do what they're *not supposed to*. We receive praise for performing well in school, inclusion when we act "cool," and affection for being agreeable. These are all subtle, everyday forms of reward. On the flip side, we might get made fun of for being different or rebelling against what's "normal." These are subtle, everyday forms of punishment. What behaviors are rewarded or punished depends a lot on where you grow up, but every society has a long list of dos and don'ts that kids pick up on as they figure out how to fit in.

The second kind of conditioning happens gradually as our beliefs are shaped by sheer repetition of experience—observing the same things occurring in association with each other over and over. For instance, whether you got good or bad grades in school, you had the endlessly repeated experience of being graded on everything. This reinforced the belief that grades are an accurate reflection of your academic abilities, which isn't actually true at all. Almost everything we consider normal seems that way to us because we've internalized the norms, rules, and conventions of our environments. Just because a belief is commonly held, that doesn't make it true. Most people might do things a certain way, but that doesn't make it the only or the best way. Conditioning doesn't offer us much of a choice, and feeling like you have no choice is a key component of healer burnout. Any amount you can wiggle free from your conditioning opens up more choices for you. So, shaking loose from your conditioning is an essential part of healing the healer. In this chapter, we'll look at a few ways our conditioning influences us.

♡ *How many of your beliefs and behaviors did you inherit without having the opportunity to decide whether or not they were right for you?*

CULTURE AND RELIGION

When I was young, my parents were not very religious. After the war and all the suffering they endured, they questioned their faith in God. But as the years passed, they followed the flow of others in their community and became more religious again. By the time I reached high school, they forced me to go to an ultra-orthodox

Jewish seminary. This was confusing for me, as I had just reached puberty and my main interest was girls.

So, I was fifteen years old at an all-boys boarding school. Everyone around me was deeply religious, praying and studying all day from 7:30 a.m. to 9:45 p.m. It was totally immersive. I did my best to fit in and act like I was interested, but I was pretending. Eventually, I found ways to literally hide—under the bed, in the closet, in the shower—and skip prayers and class. Then on weekends I'd come home, and my parents would ask, "How was it?" To which I would reply, "Great! Everything's good." And this went on for years.

I had to develop a split personality to appease my parents and conform to my environment. I knew I was living a double life, but I couldn't break their hearts after all they had been through. I couldn't tell them I was not interested in religion. I had to get away.

Eventually, a rabbi I knew got me into graduate school based on my extensive religious studies. It was a Catholic university in the United States, far away from my Canadian home. I'll never forget the first time I stepped inside the school building and saw a huge crucifix, with Jesus bleeding, on the wall. Whoa! Having had minimal exposure to the world outside of my close-knit Jewish community, I was shocked to realize Catholics also believed they were the chosen people, God's favorites. I thought, "That's crazy!" So, I started reading about Jesus and how the Jews missed the Messiah. I realized Catholics had their own interpretation of history, just like the Jews did. This was a real wake-up moment for me, which burst the bubble I had been living in. From then on, I recognized that everyone wants to feel like they are the chosen people.

The more I started traveling to other places around the world, the more I realized that perceptions of what is normal are regional. In Singapore, I once witnessed Thaipusam, a Hindu festival in which devotees pierce their cheeks, backs, and other parts of their bodies with hooks and spikes. They then go into a trance. The ritual is meant to serve as a physical sacrifice to honor the Hindu god Murugan.[1] On my first day walking down the street in Singapore, I was shocked to see people with actual meat hooks in them! Often when I'm traveling, I feel like I'm on another planet—things seem stranger than fiction. But to the people in that region, it's normal.

Religion and culture teach us what we are supposed to value and feel shame about, though it's all subjective and depends on where you live in the world. Some things are objectively true, like the Earth orbiting the sun. Other beliefs are regionally or culturally true, like the belief that Jews are the chosen people, that Jesus is the son of God, or that piercing oneself with steel hooks is an act of devotion. Most traditions people follow to this day were created thousands of years ago. Still, many consider their local beliefs objectively true; they might discriminate against those who are different or even go to war over these differences.

Having been so sheltered as a young person, I rarely spoke to non-Jewish people until my twenties. I was out of the loop when it came to fashion, sports, and pop culture. I've since joked with others who also left religious Judaism that it's like being born again at twenty years old. I had to separate myself from my orthodox conditioning to understand myself and the world around me on my own terms. This kind of exploration felt natural and necessary to me, yet it took decades to understand who I am outside of what I was taught. I had this past life, made up of tons of rules and different blessings for foods: some to be said before you eat and others for after the meal, and the prayers were different depending on what you were eating. There were hundreds of commandments to follow every day, including praying three times a day. Then all of a sudden, there were no rules, and I had no idea how to function. I felt like an animal released into the wild after twenty years in a cage.

Depending on your upbringing, you may have had to repress parts of yourself, like I did. You might carry guilt or shame for not fitting the prescribed roles others tried to put you into. It's human nature to want to belong, but we don't get to choose the families or communities we're born into. At some point, we must venture into the wild, challenge what's presented as truth, and meet ourselves on a spiritual level to learn who we really are.

I think this is what drew me to India ten times. I was fascinated by the idea of enlightenment. Enlightenment made more sense to me than any religious concept I had encountered, because it's about getting out of your mind and becoming fully present in the moment. It's not something you learn, study, or reach with age and wisdom; it's more like unlearning, a return to your original self.

Babies seem enlightened: gazing at the sky in wonder, totally present and full of wisdom. Then the baby gets older and learns that school starts at nine and bedtime is at seven, C-A-T spells *cat*, 3 + 3 = 6, and so on. There are all these things we're made to remember, which govern us as we move through life. Over time, our focus shifts from wonder and curiosity to obedience and following rules— hundreds of rules a day. The world teaches us that there are things we need to strive for to be worthy and success-ful. Enlightenment is about letting all of that go, taking a deep breath, and being present right here, right now.

It can seem almost impossible to deconstruct all the things imprinted on us by our parents, grandparents, ancestors, schools, and society. But at some point, we must question the things we have been taught and discern what is helpful and what is not helpful. We must decide which beliefs and messages to carry into the future and which ones to leave behind.

This self-inquiry is an important step in healing and finding meaning. As we open our minds and question the world around us, we find deeper meaning in ourselves. We also become more accepting of other people's beliefs and worldviews.

♥ *What were you taught about God, religion, or spirituality? What religious or cultural values were instilled in you? How about traditions? Of those values and traditions, what, if anything, feels good to you now? What does not feel good to you? Do you carry any shame as a result of how you were influenced by your culture and/or religion?*

SOCIAL EXPECTATIONS

Before founding the Institute for Integrative Nutrition, I did health and nutrition counseling. That's when I first noticed that food is a vehicle for so many other deeper issues. Pretty often, people would open up and share stories or secrets they hadn't told anyone else. Food was just the gateway.

Once, a well-educated client told me, "Yeah, I'm married. I have three daughters and a sweetheart husband, but I have a whole separate sex life on the side."

Coming from a very sheltered background, I was stunned. I couldn't believe what I was hearing. "Does your husband know?" I asked.

She said he didn't. I asked if she felt bad about it, and again, she answered no. It didn't take me long to realize that this wasn't uncommon—many people live compartmentalized double lives. They pretend to be one way while hiding a whole other side of themselves. This client was conflicted. She wanted to preserve her marriage, yet she also wanted the freedom to fulfill her desires outside of it. So, she split herself in two.

Regardless of where you come from and who you are, society has dealt you a hand of certain expectations, and these expectations dictate how you're meant to behave in order to be accepted. In American society, we are taught to work hard, get married, buy a house in the suburbs, have kids, and so on. For many, this lifestyle feels unnatural, but the need to belong is so pervasive that many people are willing to bury and sacrifice the things that set them apart. Because being an outsider is too painful and hard, they give in to the pressure to be so-called normal.

When I was forty-four and broke, my mother told me, "You're too old to be renting" and gave me money for a down payment on a house. Part of me was happy when she did this. Free money. But I also felt a sense of grief. I was basically a minimalist before it was trendy and had a real resistance to owning stuff. I felt happier when I could be light on my feet, free to travel anywhere at any time, unencumbered by possessions. I have never been the homeowning, stay-put kind of person, and I wasn't ready for the nomadic part of my life to end. I worried that owning a house would feel like a burden.

So, I got the house but didn't buy any furniture, except for a bed I bought from the previous owners. I remember feeling bothered by the electric hum of the refrigerator and other appliances, so I'd turn off the breaker switch each night to feel a little closer to nature and less like a homeowner. I figured whatever was in the fridge would stay cold until the morning. It was not a well-built home, so the wind would whistle through the walls every time it blew, connecting me to the wild in some way. That was the only time I felt at peace in that house—late at night, after I'd turned off all the electricity.

Years later, I learned the term digital nomad and finally had language for how I'd always felt. Digital nomads live a transient lifestyle and work remotely from a phone or computer as they travel. In recent years, many healers have adopted this way of living, conducting their work via video calls around the world.

Now, at seventy, I fully embrace my inner nomad, traveling as often as I can and spending time in places that feel temporary. My wandering nature, I've realized, is connected to my acceptance of impermanence. I'm not afraid to die. When you think about it, it's the most predictable thing in the world. Everyone dies, yet many people try to create illusions of permanence through the things they own. I prefer living in the moment, which feels more truthful to me. After all, we are all spiritual beings having a temporary human experience. I particularly enjoy staying at hotels for a short time because this allows me to feel anonymous. I am happiest living out of a single suitcase. As long as I have my toothbrush and a shower, I have everything I need.

Because healers are empathetic and adaptable, we are often especially good at living double lives and masking our differences to fit in to the mainstream. But suppressing our true selves causes inner conflict and prevents us from living authentically. We all have innate desires and tendencies that make us who we are, beyond what our parents, schools, and society taught us. Although society may pressure us to conform, we must have the courage to honor our individuality, even when it goes against the grain. True belonging comes not from meeting others' standards but from following our own internal compass, wherever it leads.

♡ *What social expectations did you grow up with? What was considered normal in your family and society? What were you taught about what it means to be good? Do you agree with these teachings and norms? Why or why not?*

GRIND CULTURE

We live in a culture that reveres hard work and discipline. From the time we are in school, we are taught to develop marketable skills so we can enter the workforce, contribute to society, and achieve success. As adults, it's continually instilled in us that our worth is tied to how much we are able to produce and achieve. This is especially true in big cities like New York, where there is a competitive workforce and survival-of-the-fittest mentality. This ideology surfaces in every facet of the culture, from people's work mentality to the diet industry, ultimately leading to burnout, self-sabotage, and shame.

As a result, many people struggle with expressing their emotions, cultivating healthy relationships, and setting appropriate boundaries. Trained to be cogs in the wheel of society, they lack self-awareness, self-connection, and the language to ask for what they need.

Many healers, particularly women, have internalized the idea that it's their personal responsibility to do it all, to tend to family and home while holding down a full-time job—and that if they can't hold it all together, it's a personal failure. But the truth is that no one is meant to carry the world alone. We're meant to have support systems and communities to lean on. The reason we are burned out and feel inadequate is partly because of the system we're living in.

HEALER HIGHLIGHT

"After more than fifteen years of clinical practice as a doctor, I felt emotionally crippled from pushing myself so hard, working long hours, and dealing with a lot of stress, both at work and in private. I felt completely disconnected from myself. That's when I started to study holistic wellness, which opened my eyes to the importance of self-care. Accepting my shift from doctor to patient was hugely challenging but also empowering. It gave me the courage to ask for help and receive support. Additionally, I've learned to set aside small moments of mindfulness and 'me time' every day to stay anchored in the here and now."—**CRISTIANA** from the United Kingdom

In reality, we don't need to dissociate from ourselves to be successful. What we need to thrive is help from other people, a sense of meaning, and more self-compassion. But when the majority believes that bulldozing through life is a virtue, the rest of us can't help but feel lazy or guilty when our bodies tell us we need rest. So, we continue to push ourselves, perpetuating this unhealthy cultural narrative.

Additionally, in the United States, individualism, independence, and self-reliance are heavily emphasized, unlike in countries like China, Japan, and South Korea, which hold more collectivist values. Unlike individualism, which prioritizes the rights and concerns of each individual, collectivism underscores the importance of the community. In collectivistic cultures, social rules revolve around promoting selflessness. Individuals are considered good if they are generous, helpful, dependable, and attentive to others' needs.[2]

Collectivism isn't better than individualism, or vice versa—they each have their pros and cons. But it is important to recognize how these cultural differences impact various aspects of how a society functions. China has a grind culture that rivals even that of the United States, but the focus there is on playing your part rather than trying to compete with your neighbors. As healers, our yearning to be present, to help, and to connect with others on an emotional level makes living in a grind culture an even greater challenge. Additionally, when society prioritizes individual needs, the weight on healers to uphold the collective becomes more of a burden.

♡ *How does your culture define success? Do you agree with this idea of success? Why or why not?*

OPPRESSION AND DISCRIMINATION

Unfortunately, we live in a world of inequality and injustice. Not all people have equal rights or access to education, employment opportunities, healthcare, or even basic necessities. Social hierarchies determine which groups of people within a society have more privilege than others. People oppress and discriminate against others based on race, religion, nationality, sex, sexual orientation, gender identity, socioeconomic status, age, appearance, physical and mental abilities, and countless other factors. If you are part of a marginalized group, or if you have been bullied or discriminated against in your life for any reason, you know how stressful this is. Oppression and discrimination cause traumatic injury, interfering dramatically with our self-worth and worldview.

When we grow up in environments that reinforce negative messages about who we are, we internalize those messages. We believe them. We then hold on to negative stereotypes about ourselves and accompanying feelings of inferiority, comparing ourselves with more dominant or privileged groups. Depending on which marginalized group you're in, there are a range of false messages you might have taken on without realizing it. A Black person raised in a predominantly white society may carry internalized racism and feel that they always need to prove themselves, or even prove the worthiness of their entire race. A disabled person might carry internalized ableism and question whether they have the right to request special accommodations, especially in non-disabled spaces. These are both examples of internalized oppression.

Internalized oppression often leads to feelings of shame, self-doubt, and unworthiness. It can make you doubt that you belong or lead you to believe there's something wrong with you. It can affect your self-esteem and your ability to care for yourself. It can also lead to mental health difficulties; people from marginalized groups struggle disproportionately with mental health issues. If you are constantly stressed out, on guard, and made to feel inferior to others, this will take an enormous toll on your energy and well-being.

♡ *What marginalized groups, if any, are you a part of? Do you carry shame as a result of the way society has treated you? How has this shame affected your self-worth?*

BODY IMAGE STANDARDS

Over the years, I've heard many health coaches say, "I'll be ready to take on clients when I lose twenty pounds." They are convinced they need to fit a certain mold for potential clients to take them seriously. In reality, healthy bodies come in all shapes and sizes. But we all carry some level of bias around what "healthy" looks like—especially those of us raised with specific body type ideals.

As healers, we know health is multidimensional, yet we judge ourselves by narrow beauty standards. We strive for unrealistic ideals, thinking we must embody a cookie-cutter "wellness pro" image. But health is bio-individual—we are all unique, and it is recognizing and honoring our uniqueness that is the key to health and happiness.

After I retired from IIN, my life changed pretty drastically. I had been so busy for so many years, then everything came to a stop. In my boredom, I developed some bad eating habits and began to gain weight. I began judging myself. No one else needed to judge me—I was doing it to myself. As I came to understand this, I made a decision to love myself exactly as I am, which also meant accepting my new weight. Eventually, I made peace with myself, lost the internal self-criticism, and lost the weight.

Many of us expend a lot of time and energy worrying about the size and shape of our bodies and the way we appear to others, which limits our potential. As biases around what healthy looks like persist, there may be added pressure to achieve an idealized physique for some wellness workers, like health coaches and yoga instructors, in order to walk their talk and attract clients. Our caring work is demanding as it is. The pressure to achieve an idealized physique becomes an unnecessary added source of stress, especially when we are juggling a thousand other responsibilities. When we can't attain unrealistic ideals, we become more likely to get caught up in yo-yo dieting and cycles of self-sabotage. Our self-esteem suffers as we blame ourselves for lacking self-control. Feeling self-conscious, self-critical, and ashamed, we may isolate ourselves from others.

To free ourselves from some of this excess worry and stress, it helps to acknowledge the forces at play. The diet and weight loss industry profits off people continuously striving to meet the industry's unrealistic standards. Of course, it is healthy to exercise and eat a nutritious diet—but in a way that empowers us to live our best lives possible, *not* in a way that exhausts us and keeps us down.

We are most capable of inspiring true well-being in others when we are confident and at peace in our own skin. How much energy would be freed up for our healing work if we could love our bodies as they are? When we treat our own bodies with compassion rather than criticism, we become role models, empowering others from the inside out.

♡ *In what ways are you self-critical of your body? How much of your time and emotional energy goes into trying to feel better about your appearance? If you could love your body right now, exactly as it is, how much of your energy would you free up?*

THE HEALER HIERARCHY

Despite how necessary it is to the functioning of society, caring work in the US is undervalued. A hierarchy of value exists wherein healers are valued and paid less than other members of society. Homemakers, who often double as caregivers to young children or aging parents, usually provide at least half the labor that is required to run a household, yet their work is unpaid. Home health aides, childcare providers, and other care providers offer crucial services, yet these roles—occupied mostly by women and, disproportionately, women of color—lack prestige and equitable pay (the median annual income for home health and personal aids is only $30,180).[3] Other helping professions like nursing, teaching, and social work, face a similar lack of appreciation and compensation.

Holistic practitioners also tend to rank lower in the healing hierarchy, with conventional medicine as the gold standard. Although careers in holistic health have slowly been gaining more credibility in the US, wellness workers continue to encounter skepticism. Work that is healing, intuitive, or energetic in nature is often considered less legitimate than jobs that are grounded in science or require a lot of expensive schooling.

There is a hierarchy even within the hospital system. Doctors are paid more than nurses, though nurses are usually the ones doing the heavy lifting and providing hands-on bedside care for patients. Nurses work long, grueling hours and deal with high stakes and high stress, as people's lives are on the line. They are often the ones who work the night shifts. Yet doctors get much more respect and compensation.

This hierarchy disproportionately impacts care providers who rank lower on the healer hierarchy. As a result, they frequently become discouraged or demoralized in their positions, which contributes to burnout.

♡ *Where does your work, paid or otherwise, fall in the social hierarchy? Do you ever undervalue your own contributions because of this hierarchy? Does being undervalued contribute to burnout for you?*

LIMITING BELIEFS

The combined effect of our childhood traumas and our social conditioning produces limiting beliefs: patterns that limit us from achieving our full potential. We have these tapes playing in our minds, saying, "I'm not good enough," or "I don't belong here." Many of these beliefs are unconscious. Until we identify and challenge our inner contradictions and limiting beliefs, they restrict us. They keep us from saying yes to new opportunities in spite of our soul's desire to expand, experiment, and grow.

We adopt countless false truths fed to us throughout our lives by our parents, teachers, coaches, mentors, peers, and society. But not everyone has our best interests at heart, and not everyone has the tools or self-awareness necessary to attune to us and support us the way we deserve. Other people's opinions are limited by their own motives and limited understanding of themselves, you, and the world at large. When we unconsciously accept their teachings, our brains go on autopilot. We operate under the veil of these beliefs, and that becomes our limited reality.

Some common limiting beliefs held by healers include:

- Self-sacrifice is a virtue.
- Asking for help means I am weak or lazy.
- I must be kind, generous, and attentive to others at all times.
- I am not allowed to make mistakes.
- When things go wrong, it's my fault.
- If I say no, I'm a bad [partner, sibling, coach, friend, employee, etc.].
- I'm too sensitive.
- My emotions are a burden to others.
- I am not enough.

Do any of these statements sound familiar? Have you adopted any of these beliefs as your own? Beliefs like these keep us from taking risks and speaking up for what we need. They get in the way of our ability to experience abundance, joy, confidence, and agency in our lives. They keep us from leaving relationships and jobs that no longer serve us, and from becoming the people we want to be. We carry around the beliefs we accumulate throughout our lives. That makes for a lot of baggage weighing us down.

When we live according to our past, it's like driving a car by looking in the rearview mirror. Instead of looking at the road ahead, we say, "Oh, there are three cars behind me. Maybe I should speed up." Rather than living in the present, we allow the past to dictate our future. It's like saying you dated a Scorpio once and got your heart broken, so you're never going to date a Scorpio again, or refusing to go to Chicago because you had an awful time there once as a child. As we get older and collect more and more limiting beliefs, our world keeps getting smaller. Some people get to a point where they can't even go outside without experiencing anxiety and dread. The stories we tell ourselves are powerful.

For most of us, the limiting beliefs we hold are unconscious. We limit ourselves in all kinds of ways, every day, without realizing it. It's a kind of spiritual amnesia—we forget we were once whole, complete beings. We fall for the illusion that we must conform, and we disown our deeper selves to fit in. But human beings have the unique gift of freely inventing new behaviors in ways other species can't. I always use the example of walking a dog. The dog has a habit of doing the exact same thing every day. It walks on the grass, looks for somewhere to pee, and wants to sniff everything. The dog doesn't say, "I'm going to surprise my owner today and make up stuff on the spot." But because humans have highly developed brains, we can be spontaneous. At any given moment, we might say, "You know what? This sucks. I'm going to do something totally different."

First, however, we need to uncover the deeply ingrained biases embedded in our psyche that keep us from playing big in life. We need to raise our awareness around where these beliefs originated. Then we need to unlearn the things we have been taught that are not serving us. This work is scary because it involves examining the core of who you are. But it is exciting to start following your own path.

PART III

TAKE BACK YOUR POWER

CHAPTER 6

REWRITE
YOUR STORY

♡

IN THE PREVIOUS CHAPTERS, YOU BEGAN
identifying some of the beliefs instilled in you by your
early life experiences and social conditioning. Now, it's time
to put that awareness to work. This part of the book is all
about taking back your power. What is truly in your heart
and soul, and what is just noise that's been ingrained in
you? Are you able to tell the difference? Although it takes
work, we can interrupt the patterns in our brains and reprogram the way we think. We can make the healing choice to
release the ingrained messages that we are not good enough
and replace those messages with more empowering ones.

I am going to help you rewrite the stories that no longer
serve you. To begin, create a list of the top three limiting

beliefs you are struggling with right now. These can be beliefs you've been holding on to since childhood, or they can be beliefs you are struggling with at this moment. Your limiting beliefs might be related to your career, your finances, your love life, your family, your health, or your worldview. As a tip, if you aren't sure what a limiting belief sounds like, they commonly begin with "I don't," "I can't," "I should," "I must," or "I'm not."

One healer I interviewed while writing this book, Martina, shared the following limiting beliefs with me:

1. I must be completely selfless to be a good mom.

2. I must devote all my spare time to caring for my sick dad to be a good daughter.

3. I should have a perfectly healthy marriage because I am a couples therapist.

When Martina shared these beliefs with me, I explained to her that as long as she continued to reinforce these beliefs through her thoughts and actions, they would be true. She would end up minimizing her own needs in order to be a good mom. She wouldn't be a good daughter unless she devoted all her spare time to her dad. And she'd continue to struggle with imposter syndrome as a couples therapist unless her marriage is perfect. Are these expectations realistic? No.

So, I asked Martina, "What if instead of reinforcing these beliefs, you try reframing them?"

"You mean like start telling myself the opposite?" Martina asked. "But wouldn't that be like lying to myself?"

"The point is not to lie to yourself," I explained. "Instead, you want to see if you can replace these old beliefs with beliefs that are more authentic and honest—beliefs that can guide your life in a healthier direction. For example, instead of saying, 'I must be completely selfless to be a good mom,' you might say, 'I am the mom my kids need when I take good care of myself in addition to taking care of my family.'"

"I like the sound of that," Martina said.

"Or," I continued, "instead of saying, 'I should have a perfectly healthy marriage because I am a couples therapist,' you might say, 'As a couples therapist, I am committed to showing up authentically and meeting my clients where they are.'"

Now it's your turn. Choose one limiting belief from your top three list and use the following exercise to reframe it.

1. What is your limiting belief? Write it down as a complete sentence (e.g., "I'm too old to get another degree").

2. What evidence do you have to support that this belief is *true*? For example, if your limiting belief is that you're too old to get another degree, as evidence, you might write:

    • The average grad student is in their twenties or thirties, and I'm fifty-two.

- I plan to retire within the next fifteen years.

- I am not good with technology.

3. In what ways has your limiting belief served or protected you up until this point? Write down the ways in which your belief has kept you "safe." For example:

- If I never enroll, I can't make a fool of myself or fail.

- I can avoid having a difficult conversation with my spouse.

- I don't have to worry about whether my financial investment will pay off.

4. What would your life look like if you were *not* limited by this belief? For example:

- I would talk to my spouse tonight and enroll as soon as possible.

- I would get to pursue my passion and meet new people.

- I would be able to retire without the regret of never working in the field I have always wanted to work in.

5. Finally, write down a few sentences that reframe your limiting belief in an empowering way. For example:

- I might succeed or fail, but either way, I will learn something about myself.

- It's my turn to focus on myself and do something I'm excited about.

- My age does not make me less capable of learning.

- I have access to resources and people in my network who can support me with technology if needed.

How did that exercise feel? Did anything come up that surprised you? Exercises like this can help you break old thought patterns and try on new perspectives. Use these five prompts to challenge and reframe as many limiting beliefs as you'd like. Just remember that reframing your beliefs is only the first step in taking back your power. To reinforce your new beliefs and disempower the old ones, you'll need to act according to your new beliefs. Then, in time, your reframed beliefs will become as automatic as your limiting beliefs used to be.

REPROGRAM YOUR INTERNAL OPERATING SYSTEM

When you uncover and reframe your limiting beliefs, especially the ones you have long been unconscious of, you start to reprogram your internal operating system. Your internal operating system is made up of ingrained beliefs, biases, and assumptions. It's like a lens you look through to see the world. Updating your system requires that you observe your thoughts. From there, you make a conscious effort to interrupt old thought patterns and replace them with new thoughts.

Sometimes, I like to envision thoughts like tennis balls being hit to my side of the court. I have the choice to either run after each one or let some of them bounce past me. This brings my awareness to the thoughts that serve me and the thoughts that don't, giving me the opportunity to choose only the thoughts that are going to help me play my best game.

I'll give you an example of one thing I did to update my internal operating system. For a long time, I had a habit of neglecting myself and doing things for other people to the point of exhaustion. So, I made a promise to myself that every time I did a favor for someone else, I would also do one kind thing for myself. Each time a thought came up that said, "You haven't done enough for this person. They need more help," I would interrupt the thought and replace it with, "I deserve kindness and care, too." I was able to recover a lot of my own health this way.

Your internal operating system is running a script that is mostly based on external validation. The whole system's purpose is to try to meet other people's expectations and preserve your image. And the system depends on approval from others to maintain self-esteem, safety, and identity. To update your operating system and change the thought patterns that are no longer serving you, you need to be willing to interrupt the status quo and become a leader, not a follower.

As the quotation commonly attributed to Einstein goes, "We can't solve problems with the same thinking we used to create them." In other words, you need to update your brain to expand your reality. This is not a one-time decision but an ongoing commitment to observe your thoughts, challenge them, and redirect them.

REFRAME YOUR PAST

Did you know memories are not fixed? Far from it, actually. They change over the years, morphing a little each time we recall them. Memories from long ago are especially prone to changing, so it's a good idea to not take them too literally. I don't mean to say that your memories are wrong or the things you remember never happened; rather, I mean that what actually happened matters a lot less than your *relationship* to what happened. So, if you can change your relationship to a memory, the memory changes as well. This means you have the ability to change your narrative and re-author your life. Instead of being defined by events in your past you cannot change, you can rewrite your story and reclaim your agency.

Why is reframing the past important? As children, we do the best we can to make sense of the things that happen to us, but our understanding of the world is limited. This is why we need to make a deliberate effort to update our narratives as adults, using our more sophisticated understanding of how the world works. We do this by rewriting our stories to match our current level of insight, which allows us to heal inner wounds and transform painful stories into stories of resilience.

For example, a child might develop a story that he is weak because a group of boys bullied him on the playground when he was eight years old and made him feel small. He might then carry this story into adulthood, which may cause him to feel weak around other men and not push himself hard at the gym. In this case, the man who was once a victim of bullying is allowing his eight-year-old self to run his life. Until he reframes what happened to him through an adult lens, the eight-year-old's version of the story will continue to control him.

To practice reframing, do the following exercise.

1. Try writing out a difficult experience you went through in your life. Write it the way it happened— the way it lives in you now. For example:

   When I was eight years old, I got bullied on the playground. A group of older boys surrounded me and took turns saying awful things. One boy said my arms looked like spaghetti noodles because I was so lanky. Another called me a wimpy coward. They were so cruel that they made me cry, which made me feel even weaker.

2. Now, imagine the events in your memory are playing out a short distance away from you. See if you can watch them as a bystander, with relaxed curiosity. Just observe it as an interesting episode of life happening, almost like you're an anthropologist from another planet and you simply want to see human experience in action. Watch the memory go by and pause to observe what all the people in it are feeling. Notice what it does to your sense of the memory to remain neutral about it and stay interested in it from a distance. Then rewrite your story as objectively as possible, referring to yourself in the third person. For example:

A group of older boys surround a younger boy at the playground. The older boys take turns directing insults at the younger boy based on the younger boy's size. The younger boy cries. The older boys laugh and walk away.

3. For the final part of the exercise, you're going to tell your story one more time. This time, tell it as the adult you are today. The goal is to reinterpret the event using the awareness and insight you have now. You might also create meaning from your negative experience by considering what you learned, how it shaped you for the better, and what positive values you developed as a result. For example:

A group of older boys picked on me when I was eight years old because I was smaller than them. Kids can be cruel. I wonder if the bullies had trouble in their homes that caused them to act out. Or maybe they were being guided to target me by peer pressure. Either way, the bullies probably lacked nurturing. Because I was bullied as a kid, I go out of my way to be kind to people. Rather than judge others for their shortcomings, I try to remain curious and open. I am a good protector of others and myself. To me, being a strong man is about taking care of others, not causing others pain.

How did that exercise feel? Do you see how the practice of witnessing past events objectively and applying mature emotions to childhood memories can recast those memories? You should go through this series of questions at your own pace and rewrite as many stories from your past as you want. It is only out of habit that we allow emotions from the past to color our memories of past events. We also have the option of allowing our present emotions to color and interpret the past. The more awareness and mature insight you bring to your interpretation of past experiences, the more control you will have over your future.

As we gain more awareness, we can also reframe ongoing struggles. If you're anything like me, your life might be colored by feeling like an outsider. Some of us highly sensitive, empathic types carry shame around not being able to assimilate into the world the way other people do. If this is your story, you can rewrite it with more compassion for yourself now that you are aware of this personality trait: you weren't defective as a child, just sensitive in a way that most people aren't. See if you can reframe some past experiences through the lens of being highly sensitive, noting that much of society isn't set up to support people who feel deeply.

Remember, rewriting your personal narrative is an ongoing practice. But over time, reframing past experiences will help you develop more self-compassion and move beyond difficult emotions and limiting beliefs. The stories we tell ourselves shape our identity and create our reality. As you practice reframing old narratives, you will also learn to approach future challenges with more optimism and curiosity.

♡ *Are you still telling yourself old stories developed in childhood about who you are? How would your life be different if you updated these stories into more empowering narratives?*

CHAPTER 7

HEAL YOUR CHILDHOOD WOUNDS

♡

YOUR PAST HAS MADE YOU WHO YOU ARE today, but it doesn't have to define who you'll become tomorrow. We've been talking about the past in terms of childhood wounds, developmental trauma, and conditioning. But the past, of course, doesn't really exist. Memories exist as patterns in our neural networks. Unresolved emotions exist as patterns of tension in our bodies. We carry memories and emotions around in the present, and we can learn to release them to make our futures lighter.

So, how can you tell whether a wound from the past needs healing? One clue is getting triggered when something happening in the present reminds you of something from your past. Suddenly, the past feels as if it's happening again, right now. Old feelings return, and you resort to old behaviors for managing those feelings. Most of the time when this happens, you don't even know you've been triggered; you just feel upset, anxious, down, embarrassed, defensive, or aggressive. You might not know why you feel that way. And you might think the feelings are about what's going on in the here and now.

Through the process of healing, you will become less and less prone to being triggered. You won't go around confusing the present with the past as often. Instead of having an automatic reaction to events, you'll choose how you want to respond to them. Much of the time, you can even choose how you feel.

Healing often seems like a mysterious process, but it isn't. It requires courage to face your memories and feel your feelings. It also requires some assistance from other people. Let's talk about the steps involved in healing. Then we'll talk about resilience, which is one of the great benefits of overcoming painful experiences, and something you can deliberately cultivate in yourself.

FIND PARTNERS IN HEALING

I can't emphasize this enough: you cannot heal all alone. Much of the hurt experienced in early life happens in the context of relationships. Other people hurt you or didn't meet your needs, or you had to do things that weren't right for you to make other people happy, to protect yourself from them, or to belong. Maybe you feared someone or lost someone, or other people excluded, shamed, or ignored you. Of course, there are hurts that aren't interpersonal in nature. But if you weren't able to spontaneously heal from those hurts after they happened, it's probably because the people around you didn't know how to help you or discouraged you from feeling what you needed to feel to properly process that pain. Healing is either supported or hindered by other people.

Just as we have a basic human drive for connection, we instinctively know that we need other people in order to heal. When you experienced difficulties in your youth, it would have made all the difference if someone was really there for you. Imagine what it would have been like if you'd had a real ally—someone who got what it was like for you, who listened to you and loved you and made room for your feelings, who helped you sort through confusion and recover from shock. Regardless of whether or not you had that kind of support back then, you can have it now. Allowing someone to be your partner in healing helps complete a cycle that started back when you were trying to manage a hurt on your own.

As the primary teacher at IIN, I spent a lot of time teaching small groups and large audiences alike, and I continue to teach now that I've retired. Whenever I teach a group in person, I devote a lot of time to paired sharing. For example, if I'm talking about the importance of finding partners in healing, I might say, "Turn to the person next to you and tell them about an experience you had recently when you could have used support." I do this because I have always believed that people learn as much from one another as they do from me or any other teacher on the stage. Rather than me lecturing down to people, I want them to open up and share what's in their hearts, make connections, and realize they are not alone in what they are going through.

Although professional counseling or therapy can be invaluable in working through painful experiences and childhood wounds, there is also tremendous therapeutic value in partnering with others who get what we're going through (e.g., fellow healers).

In my decades of teaching, I have seen firsthand how powerfully healing peer support can be. When we open up and share vulnerably, and when we listen with empathy instead of judgment, we help shoulder each other's burdens.

One effective way to find healing partners is to intentionally carve out time to support one another through deep listening.

Here are some suggestions for how to practice peer support:

- Schedule and prioritize intentional time with a fellow healer. This could be weekly, monthly, or however frequently you desire.

- In these sessions, take turns sharing and listening to each other. Ideally, you'll refrain from giving advice or trying to fix the other person. Instead, emphasize listening with empathy, making room for the other person's feelings, and keeping an open, curious mind.

- You don't need to be an expert who knows exactly where to guide someone. You just need to hold their hand and be on the journey with them. It's a collaboration.

Because we all have blind spots, we need other people to reflect back to us what they hear when we describe our emotions. Our programming determines how we experience reality. We're often too immersed in our own stories to see ourselves objectively. It can be helpful to invite others to witness us in our process and share their perspectives. This doesn't have to be a one-on-one experience; we also heal in support groups and growth-oriented communities.

The instinct to seek partners in healing is stronger than most people realize. Even when we don't do it consciously, we unconsciously draw people to us that we intuitively sense can help. One common way we seek healing is through the people we choose as romantic partners. We seek out love relationships with people who remind us of our parents or primary caretakers. Then, often without being aware of it, we project our past wounds onto them, trying to provoke specific responses from them. We're unconsciously trying to get triggered, trying to feel the same unresolved feelings from old hurtful experiences, hoping this time there will be someone there for us who loves us. It's as if we harbor some hope that things will be different this time around, thereby resolving some unfinished business from childhood. Unfortunately, this rarely works. Most of the time, you just end up with two triggered people competing with each other for attention and understanding.

Relationships in which both partners consciously commit to working on their underlying issues together can be healing and transformative. But it's also a lot to expect of a romantic partner, who is so invested in the outcome. So, I suggest setting up healing partnerships with less pressure and lower stakes, like with friends, family members, or other healing partners.

💙 *Do you have healing partners in your life already? If not, are there people you might want to establish such a partnership with?*

EXTRACT THE PAST FROM THE PRESENT

Let's talk for a moment about what it means to be triggered. It's a good metaphor. Imagine you're walking around with a loaded gun. The safety is off, and your finger is already lightly squeezing the trigger. Then someone unexpectedly comes around the corner, startling you, and the gun goes off. You wouldn't say, "How dare that person make me shoot that gun! I would never have fired it if they had warned me they were coming around the corner." It would be obvious that their role in the gun going off was minimal. You were a firearm accident waiting to happen!

Emotional triggers are the same. Something happens, and you are suddenly under the sway of a powerful emotion. It seems like the current event caused the emotion, but that emotion was preloaded within you. It was lying dormant, waiting for the right stimulus to release it. But realizing this can be tricky, especially when the triggering event is another person. The important thing to do in these moments is to recognize why you are triggered—and the reason is almost always the same: something in the present reminds you of something unresolved from your past.

For instance, if someone speaks in an angry tone, you might feel scared like you did when that happened to you as a child. You might feel powerless and find yourself doing anything you can to fix it, because that's what you did when you were young. Unhealed childhood wounds rob us of our power to think and react according to our highest truth. Old feelings take over. Then old behaviors take over, and in that moment, they seem like your only option for dealing with the present situation.

But let's say you are aware that hearing someone speak in an angry tone is triggering for you. That awareness empowers you to act differently. Sure, the angry person might be out of line, but instead of responding in a reactive manner, you can thoughtfully decide how to respond in a way that aligns with your values.

So, how do you stop being triggered? You learn to distinguish between the present and the past.

For this next exercise, you'll work with a personal experience of being triggered. You can wait until something happens that triggers you, or you can think back to a recent moment when you were triggered. To begin, acknowledge that you've been triggered and try to identify all the parts of the triggering experience. What happened to trigger you? What feelings did you feel as a result? What did you notice yourself doing in response to the feelings?

Use this awareness as a launching point, then complete the next three parts of this exercise.

First, ask yourself, "What from my past does this current experience remind me of?" You might be able to recall many past experiences similar to this one. Choose one from as early in your life as you can remember. Let's use the previous example of someone speaking in an angry tone leading to you feeling scared and scrambling to fix the situation. You might, for instance, recall a moment from childhood when your father got furiously angry at you.

For the second part of the exercise, try to find three ways the past and present events are similar to each other and three ways they are different. Here's an example:

Three Similarities

1. My father got angry out of nowhere, surprising me, and the person in the present also suddenly switched to an angry tone of voice.

2. My father was older than me, and this person is also older than me.

3. In my memory, my father was yelling at me at night, and I was tired. I'm tired now, too, from not getting enough sleep.

Three Differences

1. My father was a man, and the person in the present is a woman.

2. As a child, there was nowhere I could go to escape. Now, I am independent and even have a car. I am free to leave if I want.

3. When I was scared as a child, the feelings were overpowering. Now, I know how to breathe and calm my anxiety, as long as I remember to do so.

This exercise may seem simple, but it can be very powerful. By recognizing these similarities and differences, you become more self-aware and empowered to handle the triggering event. You can see that your current feelings come from something in the past, and you can tell that what's happening now really isn't the same as what happened then. Crucially, some points can almost always be included in your list of differences; as a child, you had limited resources, information, and options, whereas now, you're older and have many resources to draw on, far more information, and plenty of options. Maybe the most important difference is that you now have partners in healing—caring about you, listening, and offering support.

In the next part of the book, we'll identify the resources you have available to you in your life now and figure out how to get more of the ones you lack. Your ability to develop inner resources and access outer resources makes your life now remarkably different from your life back then.

The third part of this exercise is where things get interesting. To prove to yourself that the past is not happening now, find a way to respond to the present situation that's the opposite of how you responded in the past. If, in the past, you responded to someone speaking in an angry tone of voice by becoming submissive and trying desperately to calm them down, there are many creative ways you could react differently now. You could, for instance, say to them, "Hold on a second," rush out as if you just remembered something, and then not come back. If they ask you about it later, you can say you have a very low tolerance for angry communication. Or rather than thinking angry tones are bad and dangerous, you could join them and shout back: "Now we're speaking to each other in our angry voices!" Or you might simply calm your system with some deep breaths and say nothing at all, allowing the other person to have their feelings without doing anything to fix the situation.

You don't need to try any of these alternate responses in the heat of the moment. Instead, you can call up your healing partner later on and role-play to experiment with what it would feel like to defy your patterned trigger response. It might feel uncomfortable for you to break those patterns, even within the safety of a healing partnership. You might even have strong emotions come up for you. That's usually a good sign. It means you are stepping into your power after feeling powerless for a long time.

At one point in my life, I was healing some of the generational trauma I inherited from my family. Without realizing it, I had come to feel like life was a prison, like I was trapped by fear and couldn't make a move. Some friends I did peer counseling with suggested a process for me to experiment with behaving opposite to the way I usually would when triggered. They covered me in a pile of pillows and chairs, whatever was around, to literally trap me. Then I smashed my way out of my pillow prison, yelling and declaring my freedom. After we did this a few times, feelings came up. I allowed myself to experience them, and I felt much freer afterward. Even though healing involves facing difficult emotions, the process can be fun and empowering.

Of course, there are going to be times when you feel a wave of guilt, desperation, shame, powerlessness, confusion, or frustration, and you're not going to be able to trace the feeling back to a specific experience in your past. That's okay. All you need to do is pause and recognize what you're experiencing. Simply notice what you're feeling, remain curious and open, and go from there.

♥ *Can you recognize when you're triggered? Can you identify feelings that come up frequently for you that might have originated in your past? Can you imagine what it would be like if you were no longer triggered in those ways and plagued by those feelings?*

LET FEELINGS DO THEIR THING

For better or worse, it's not possible to think your way to healing. Emotional release—feeling your feelings—is an essential part of the healing process. If you feel sadness as a gloomy cloud hovering over you, that's very different from actively crying and releasing the sadness. When someone close to you dies, for instance, crying is a necessary part of grieving. If you're not able to cry, the sadness gets trapped or repressed, thereafter continuing to color your experience.

When we're hurt, feelings spontaneously spring up. If we allow those feelings to do their thing, they pass through us like waves. A wave of grief will fill the body with sadness until it overflows in tears. The tears help to release and process the experience of hurt. Crying, laughing, screaming, shaking, making sounds, and freaking out are all ways that emotions move through us. We're often reluctant to allow these natural processes to occur because we try to avoid painful emotions. The irony of this is that when you let feelings do their thing, release doesn't take very long, whereas if you repress or resist those feelings, they can hang around for the rest of your life. To feel better in the long term, you need to be willing to feel bad in the short term.

Some people don't have easy access to their feelings. In many cultures, people of all genders are taught from a young age that openly expressing emotions is unacceptable. Men, in particular, often learn that they shouldn't cry, show fear, or express any emotion besides anger. This robs people of their ability to heal, which requires experiencing the full spectrum of emotions. This is why having partners in healing can be so helpful. They help create a safe space to feel feelings and encourage you to express emotions without judgment. Learning to access emotions through the body is a process. Sometimes, we need help identifying what we're feeling so we can give language to it first. Then we can direct our awareness to where we sense the emotions in our body. Labeling feelings and identifying their somatic components are basic steps to develop emotional intelligence.

One of the most effective ways to access your feelings is through the exercise I described earlier. When you behave in ways that are the opposite of your old, triggered behavior patterns, repressed feelings may surface; that's one way you know you're on the right track. Some people are overwhelmed by their feelings much of the time. If that's true for you or someone you're helping, the goal is not to completely release every emotion all at once. Instead, you want to try slowing down the process of feeling. Focus on the fact that you're safe in the present. If you're working with a client or a patient, remind them that nothing bad is happening now, and that they're not alone because you're with them. Slowing down helps us move through emotions without being flooded by them.

When feelings are given the opportunity to move through, be expressed, and release themselves, something pretty cool happens: people spontaneously begin to have insights. Unprocessed emotions make for poorly understood experiences. It is as if the trapped feelings are interfering with our ability to think clearly in the areas where we've been hurt. Once the feelings shift, your adult mind can think more clearly and make sense of things that didn't make sense when you were younger.

This is a key point about healing. Its goal is not to return to what you were like before you were hurt. The goal of healing is to become a new version of you, one that has learned from the past and grown in the process, thereby becoming less vulnerable to being hurt in the same ways again. The more you practice leaning into difficult emotions rather than avoiding them, the more resilient, mature, and compassionate toward yourself and others you will become.

♥ *How comfortable are you with allowing yourself to feel your feelings? Do you need more practice? Do you need support to slow down those feelings so you're not flooded by them?*

RELEASE TRAUMA STORED IN THE BODY

Just as it is important to move emotions through our bodies by practicing various forms of emotional release, it is also important to move physical stress and tension through the body. Activities like bodywork, massage, yoga, dance, sports, or other physical exercise can help release chronic tightness or pain. When you're taking on a complex problem like healing wounds from childhood, it's best to approach it holistically and from multiple angles. You can use cognitive reframing to reshape old stories, practice emotional release to express feelings, and use physical release through movement or bodywork to unwind long-held bodily tension. Addressing mental, emotional, and physical layers together creates an integrated approach for healing.

HEALER HIGHLIGHT

"Before the pandemic, I began caring for my elderly mother who lives an hour away because she refused other help. It turned into four-hour commutes one to four times a week and eight- to twelve-hour days, forcing me to put my career as a social worker on hold. My son was also in crisis, so I was giving twenty-four hours a day to two loved ones in serious need. We had many traumatic events, made worse by COVID because accessing services was nonexistent. My own health crashed. My mom was eventually diagnosed with Alzheimer's but refused to leave her home, before passing away last October. I am just now starting to get my nervous system calmed down from the trauma, even though I've been focused on healing full time for over a year, seeing practitioners and on intensive protocols to heal."—**MAUREEN** from Vermont

Traumatic experiences provoke animal reactions in the body: fight, flight, and freeze responses. When the energy activated by these instincts remains trapped in the nervous system, trauma-specific residues are left behind. Sometimes it's stress that lives deep in muscular holding patterns. Sometimes it's a dysregulated nervous system prone to hyperarousal or dissociation. Somatic interventions focus on interrupting habitual patterns stored in the body and discharging tension.

In graduate school, I had a psychology professor who said, "You can't change a person's psychology without changing where they hold their psychology in their body." He then introduced me to Rolfing, a form of bodywork that reorganizes the body's connective tissues, also called fascia. Rolfing is similar to massage but more intense. It focuses on releasing, realigning, and balancing the whole body and creating structural changes.[1]

The first time I tried Rolfing, it broke me wide open. It was as if this tightly wound structure created around my life, who I am, and where I hold my reservoirs of energy and tension evaporated overnight. I became a blank slate again—tabula rasa. Bodywork helps move tension through and out of the body. To this day, whenever I get a really good massage, it's like hitting the reset button. Afterward, I feel more grounded and renewed.

The kind of bodywork that breaks down structure isn't right for everyone, though. Some of us need to build up a sense of internal structure instead. Developing core strength can be paradigm-shifting for someone who has never felt that kind of internal stability. Yoga that emphasizes strengthening as much as flexibility can have a similar effect. Whether you're breaking down muscular armoring or building up structure, when you're working to overcome childhood wounds, don't leave your body behind!

♥ *Are there patterns of chronic tension you carry in your body that might be residues from trauma in your past? Have you experienced what it's like to free up those holding patterns?*

FORGIVE THOSE WHO HAVE HURT YOU

Another key tool to heal your past is through compassion. With compassion, we're able to forgive those who have hurt us.

Everyone is always doing the best they can with what they've got. Sometimes what they've got is a lot of hurt they're carrying around, like you. Also like you, they may be lacking skills or resources, and that limits what they're capable of. If you can really get inside someone else's experience and imagine walking in their shoes, you'll realize that they are compelled to act as they do by internal pressures and external constraints. This is true of everyone in your personal history. That's the heart of compassion—understanding that everyone is doing their best with what they've been given, even when they hurt others. At our core, no one really wants to hurt anyone else, but we do it all the time anyway.

When you bring your adult sense of compassion to the characters in your memories, you have the option of forgiving those people. Forgiveness helps us move on from the pain of the past and can improve our mental and physical health. If you're holding a grudge against someone who hurt you, you have the power to forgive them for your own sake. There's a Buddhist saying that illustrates this concept: "Holding on to anger is like grasping a hot coal with the intent of throwing it at someone else; you are the one who gets burned."

To begin the process of forgiveness, it's important to acknowledge for yourself what hurt you. Do this in your mind, on paper, or in conversation with a healing partner. Then, make the conscious decision to forgive whoever hurt you and let go of any resentment. You don't need to have a conversation with the person who hurt you. This process is more about you than them. Forgiveness can happen inside your own heart even while you are alone.

To forgive, you don't need to accept that what the offender did to hurt you was okay; you only need to accept that it happened and commit to moving on. If you can find a silver lining in the situation, that's even better. Maybe you learned something in the process of getting hurt that helped you grow. Or maybe you are now better equipped to know what you need and want for yourself moving forward. This knowledge can provide additional relief.

It might be hard at first to generate compassion for those who hurt you, but letting go of that burning coal of negative emotions will be healing and powerful. It may also help you feel more in control and less stuck.

💗 *Who have you forgiven from your past? Who would you like to forgive, even if it feels too daunting to imagine right now?*

RESOLVE THE PAST

The past is finite. There's only so much of it to put behind you. There are only so many childhood wounds to overcome. If you're new to the idea of healing from your past, beginning the process can feel overwhelming, as if the past just goes on and on. But it doesn't go on and on. The past only feels endless when you don't heal and continue to repeat the same patterns over and over. Once you really commit to healing, it's possible to work your way through all the major pain points from your life story. The reward is a refreshingly open-ended future, free of all those lingering aches from long ago.

💗 *What do you imagine it might be like to go forward into a wide-open future, unburdened by your personal history?*

DEVELOPING RESILIENCE

One benefit of healing childhood wounds is that we become more resilient. Growing up with chaos, abuse, neglect, or other traumas causes our stress response systems to become dysregulated. We may shut down or become overwhelmed when we experience familiar stressors as adults. Overcoming these hardships, however, makes us far more capable than we would have been if life had always been easy and comfortable.

HEALER HIGHLIGHT

"As a holistic lifestyle and nutrition coach, I started conducting virtual coaching sessions during the COVID-19 pandemic and felt that my services were needed badly. My clients appreciated me taking care of both their physical and emotional well-being. Some even praised me for changing their lives. But I struggled privately after my father and brother passed away weeks apart. To keep moving forward and sustain my clients, I had to rapidly learn new coping skills, drawing on inner resilience and strength."—**SABEEN** from Pakistan

When you think of the word *resilience*, what comes to mind? People with a lot of resilience have a high threshold for stress, so they're able to adapt, overcome, and recover from it efficiently. The more resilient you are, the more equipped you'll be to face new challenges and see possibilities inside of difficult situations. You'll bounce back faster, so stress will be less likely to accumulate, and you'll be less likely to experience burnout.

Resilience is *not* the same thing as dissociation or denial. Many people appear resilient because they are disconnected from themselves and therefore able to push themselves to superhuman limits, at least temporarily. But abandoning oneself to cope is not an efficient way to handle stress. It won't lead to happiness, even if it leads to superficial success. The way to build authentic resilience is by actually dealing with our stuff.

Research shows caregiving can take a toll on physical and mental health. But some caregivers experience fewer negative effects than others because they are more resilient.[2] This applies to wellness workers as well. We all have different life experiences that shape our ability to overcome challenges. Those who develop inner resources early on tend to be more resilient. They are less burdened by trauma and bounce back quicker from challenging situations. Even if you didn't develop inner resources early on, you can cultivate resilience now. Here are some tips for increasing resilience as a healer.

Build a Support Network

Resilience is not only something we cultivate as individuals; it's something we can build on a collective level by connecting with people who make us feel supported and understood. By seeking out meaningful social connections and avoiding social isolation, we increase our resilience and improve our emotional well-being. Knowing we can rely on the support of people we trust makes challenging situations easier to manage. I talk more about the healing power of community support in chapter 13.

♥ *Who is in your support network now? Are there others you'd like to include?*

Step Out of Your Comfort Zone

Another way to build resilience is by gradually exposing yourself to things that challenge your comfort zone. Taking risks has the compounding effect of making you stronger over time. For example, if you have a fear of dancing in public, you might try learning a dance routine by yourself in the mirror. Once you gain some confidence, you could join a fitness dance class in your area. Eventually, you might even build up enough resilience to dance freestyle at your cousin's wedding. Every time you step out of your comfort zone and prevail, your body gets the message that what you once feared isn't so scary after all.

♥ *How have you already grown by stretching outside your comfort zone? What kinds of risks remain the most challenging for you to take on?*

Practice Being Kind to Yourself

Self-compassion is an important aspect of resilience because it is easier to go through difficult experiences with someone kind and loving than someone critical and judgmental. When you can be that kind and loving person to yourself, life's challenges feel less daunting. When you create an environment of safety within yourself, you build resilience while reducing stress and anxiety.

Research psychologist Kristin Neff found that the number one reason people are self-critical is because they believe if they are too kind to themselves, they will become self-indulgent and lazy. They think they need the harsh voice of self-criticism to keep them motivated.[3] But actually, the opposite is true. The more we engage in self-criticism, the more we stress ourselves out and shut ourselves down. To function at our best, we need to be able to treat ourselves with kindness, especially during difficult times.

A great way to practice being more compassionate toward yourself is to get in the habit of treating yourself the way you would treat a dear friend: with kindness, encouragement, empathy, and patience. Self-compassion is about putting aside perfectionism, embracing your flaws, and observing your feelings without judgment or shame.

The way we treat ourselves also affects how we treat others. When we are self-critical, we are more critical toward others. So, practicing self-compassion might be the most important thing you do to create a better world.

♡ *In which ways are you already strong in self-compassion? In which areas are you still self-critical?*

Practice Mindfulness

Staying rooted in the present moment through mindfulness allows us to face tough times without getting panicked and overwhelmed. A key component of mindfulness is the capacity to witness. If you can watch your thoughts and feelings come and go, you'll train your brain over time to understand that you are not your thoughts and feelings—you are the observer watching them. Thoughts and feelings endlessly shift and change, but the watcher remains constant. Cultivating your capacity to witness puts space between what you feel and how you choose to respond to it. Having that gap makes all the difference. Instead of reacting immediately, you bring your attention to what is happening for you internally and then choose how you wish to respond externally.

Another important aspect of mindfulness is expanded awareness. As you come to identify yourself less with your thoughts and feelings, you'll become less self-concerned and nearsighted. You'll be able to take in more, broadening your field of awareness. This makes it easier to keep perspective and make clear-headed decisions. Meditation is the means most people use to practice mindfulness, but that doesn't need to mean closing your eyes and sitting still; you are meditating any time you breathe with awareness, slow down, and bring your attention to the present moment.

♡ *Can you bring yourself to the present moment— nowhere to go and nothing to do—right now?*

Shift Your Expectations

Suffering is strongly linked to our expectations and the stories we tell ourselves.[4] This is not to say you should dismiss all your negative emotions or try to convince yourself that your situation isn't challenging. However, sometimes we get stuck in the mindset that life is simply supposed to be a certain way. We may carry the belief, for instance, that all clients or patients should be easy to work with, or that our caregiving responsibilities are unfair. Here is where we have the power to shift our perspective. Life, in fact, is not always fair. Clients and patients may be challenging to work with for many reasons. And caregiving is a very common role. In fact, it's estimated that over half of Americans over the age of fifty are caregivers, and this number is expected to keep rising as the aging population increases. Regardless of how your life may change, it is possible to adjust your outlook and expectations. Instead of dwelling on what your life could or "should" have looked like, try accepting and focusing on what is.

The goal with each of these resilience-building strategies is to get you better equipped to face challenges and stressors as they arise. The more you practice these skills, the more safety and wholeness you will feel on a daily basis, whether times are tough or not. After all, resilience is not only something you reach for in "break glass in case of emergency" situations. It's a well of internal strength you can pull from as often as you need to. Resilience will help you to take better care of yourself and navigate life's everyday challenges with a greater sense of ease.

To complete this section, I invite you to try the following exercise, which will help you connect with your inner strengths and resources. This exercise is inspired by the strength-based approach in positive psychology, which focuses on human potential rather than weaknesses and flaws.[7]

1. Name a significant obstacle you have overcome in your life. I suggest going with the first thing that comes to mind.

2. How did you overcome it? What skills and strengths did it require (e.g., patience, creativity, determination)?

3. What resources or people helped you? Whom or what did you rely on for support?

4. How can you use those strengths, skills, and resources to overcome a current challenge you are facing?

CHAPTER 8

ASSERT YOUR BOUNDARIES

♡

WE ARE BORN KNOWING WHEN WE NEED something. Babies cry when they are hungry, scared, or need their diaper changed. They may not have the language to articulate what they need in words, but they make it known in one way or another. But as we grow older, we are taught to hide our needs—to be disciplined, polite, and appropriate, and to avoid inconveniencing others. How many times have you heard a parent say, "You're fine," to a crying child? Maybe the child isn't fine and they need someone to validate what they're feeling, not dismiss it.

Over time, many of us learn to repress our emotions and stop advocating for ourselves. This is a problem because when we lose touch with ourselves and stop trusting our gut to tell us what we need, it diminishes our ability to form truly authentic relationships. We may become more anxious in social situations because we lack the defenses to protect our boundaries from being crossed. We may lack the language, skills, or courage to express our needs. We may end up saying yes to things we don't want to do instead of standing up for ourselves, then harbor resentment over it.

Healers and caregivers often find it especially challenging to set boundaries because we work intimately with others. Our empathic nature can make it difficult to say no or set limits, even when we are exhausted and overwhelmed. This is particularly difficult for those attuned to seeking out and helping wounded people. Many healers struggle with guilt over feeling selfish when we aren't available to assist people in need, as caring for others provides purpose and meaning. Without proper boundaries, healers risk facing burnout, resentment, and compassion fatigue. It's essential for us to balance helping others with self-care so we can sustain ourselves.

Setting boundaries means consistently communicating your needs and preferences: what you want and don't want, what works for you and what doesn't. If everyone did this well, we'd all get along better.

Unfortunately, it's not always as simple as that. Setting boundaries can be uncomfortable, especially if you are used to allowing other people to direct your time and energy. In this chapter, I cover the ins and outs of boundaries so that you will be better equipped to set them with ease.

HEALER HIGHLIGHT

"As a transformation coach, consultant, and teacher, I've learned that striking a balance between giving to others and caring for yourself means knowing yourself and your limits, and setting boundaries where needed. But the idea of harmony resonates more with me than balance. Sometimes, we give more and have less time for self-care. It's not balanced, but there is harmony. And sometimes, we step back, help others less, and tend to ourselves—also harmony. It's about adapting to find that holy, harmonious flow."—JOSHUA from Washington

BOUNDARIES ARE BRIDGES

Some people think of boundaries like barriers, but I prefer to think of them as bridges. The purpose of setting an interpersonal boundary is to protect your mental, emotional, and physical well-being. When you let another person know, "This is who I am, and this is what I need to feel respected and balanced," you are inviting them to see and honor the real you. You are letting them in on what you need to thrive, which is a kind of intimacy, when you think about it. It's also a way of demonstrating that you have self-awareness and self-worth.

What most healers find challenging about asserting boundaries is risking the possibility of looking bad, seeming mean, or hurting other people's feelings. This is especially true for people pleasers who try very hard not to upset anyone around them. It is natural for us humans to want to be liked. It is also natural to fear losing relationships with people we care about over speaking our truth. But when we aren't willing to disappoint others, we inevitably end up disappointing ourselves.

The good news is that it is possible to be an authentically nice person who is genuinely supportive of others while still looking after your own needs. But this doesn't mean you can control how other people react to your needs—you can't. Inevitably, you are going to encounter people who get upset by your boundaries or challenge them, which will give you useful information about these people and your relationships. And if you lose any relationships over speaking up and asking for what you need, they probably weren't serving you in the first place.

Although taking a step back from certain relationships and saying no to things you don't want to do can be uncomfortable, keep in mind that whenever you say no to something, you are saying yes to something else. For example, saying no to a friend who drains all your energy creates space for a new friend who is a better energetic match for you to enter your life. Saying no to attending a party on a Friday night after a long workweek means saying yes to spending a few hours reading and recharging in the comfort of your home.

Although it might sound oxymoronic, daring to live a life with boundaries is liberating and rewarding. When you set healthy limits for yourself, your confidence and self-esteem will improve. Your life will feel simpler, you'll have more free time to do the things you want, and your relationships will become more fulfilling because they'll be honest.

STRENGTHENING INNER BOUNDARIES

To some extent, boundaries are an inside job. Do you have a firm sense of where you end and others begin? Or do you tend to merge emotionally with others and take on what they seem to be feeling? Do you have a sense of your personal space? Can you tell when someone crosses into it? When it comes to connecting with others, are you able to control when you let people in or shut them out emotionally and energetically? Just as our skin forms a literal protective boundary around our physical bodies, we each have an intuitive sense of emotional and energetic boundaries around our inner selves. This personal space allows us to engage safely and comfortably with others, while withdrawing when we feel intruded upon. Learning to set clear interpersonal boundaries helps ensure mutual understanding and respect.

Having a well-developed inner sense of your physical, energetic, emotional, and personal space makes the process of establishing and maintaining interpersonal boundaries much easier. So, before we talk about strategies for asserting outer boundaries with others, I want to walk you through a series of brief exercises for strengthening your sense of inner boundaries. Doing these with a healing partner is ideal. Your partner doesn't need to do anything except be there. These exercises are all about you sensing your own boundaries. If you don't have another person with you, you can be your own partner by sitting in front of a mirror.

For the first exercise, sit on the floor facing your partner. Draw an imaginary circle around yourself on the ground. You can even use a piece of string to make a visible circle, if you like. Your partner should be outside the circle. Now see if you can focus your attention inward and become aware of the physical boundaries of your body occupying the space within the circle. Imagine your body emanating energy to fill the circle so that the edges push up against its boundaries. What sensations arise as you give yourself permission to fully inhabit this space? What thoughts or emotions surface as you experience yourself as a separate entity from your partner? Can you grant them freedom to just be, without taking on their emotions as your own? The goal here is to feel grounded in your body, take up space unapologetically, and notice what it's like to separate emotionally from someone else. This alone can feel strange at first. See if you can tune in to the specific emotions and physical sensations alive within you in the moment, accepting them without judgment. Consider that your partner likely feels their own distinct emotions separate from yours. Allow those to coexist without adopting them as your own.

For the next exercise, put your hands up in front of you with your palms facing your chest. Tap your chest with your fingertips and say the word *me*. Do it a couple of times: "Me . . . me." Now, turn your palms outward toward your partner and make a pushing away motion. Do this a few times while saying out loud, "Not me . . . not me." That's the whole exercise. Go back and forth between *me* and *not me* with the accompanying gestures. All you need to do is make this distinction and notice how it feels. You are the person you're tapping, and the other person, whoever they may be, is not you.

Until you actually try this, it may sound silly. But for some people, curious things happen when they make these simple statements and motions; it's not uncommon for people to feel guilty just for acknowledging that the other person isn't them. Once you've tried this one-on-one with someone, you can do it anywhere. Outside in a crowded place, you can subtly make the motions with your hands while subvocalizing the words to yourself. You are only you—no one else!

Here's a simple exercise to feel your body's boundary more distinctly. Start by sitting cross-legged on the floor, either facing a partner or by yourself. Cup your hands under your knees and pull upward while simultaneously pushing your knees down against your hands. The tension between the two forces will activate your abdominal muscles. You can also do this exercise sitting in a chair by putting your feet firmly on the ground and placing your hands, palms up, under your thighs, then pulling up with your hands while pushing down with your legs. This should make you sit up very straight and sense your abs working. Feel what it's like to have the front of your body be solid. Can you sense a real physical barrier protecting the vulnerable parts of your body? Can you allow that barrier to be strong? Now picture various people in your life in front of you. If you have a real partner with you, project those people onto your partner. Notice what it's like to have a strong barrier dividing you from each person you visualize. You might include people you feel unsure about, those who tend to dominate you, and people you have complicated relationships with. When you have a strong front, is there any difference in your experience of these visualized people? Believe it or not, a strong abdominal core strengthens your sense of boundedness.

For the final exercise, face your partner (real or imaginary) and say something you're afraid might disappoint them. This isn't about the specific person in front of you, as they're just acting as a stand-in. It's best if you make your statement as simple as possible. For example, try simply saying, "No." Other things you can experiment with saying are, "I said no," "No, thank you," "Not anymore," "Not going to happen," "I'm not interested," "I can't," "I won't," or "I'm sorry" (with the implication that you're apologizing for disappointing them). As in the previous exercises, notice the feeling that comes up around disappointing the other person. Is it difficult to tolerate? Try to stick with that challenging emotion. Take some breaths. If you need to, activate your abs. Allow the other person to be disappointed and yourself to have whatever feeling arises in you as a result. The capacity to tolerate that feeling is a prerequisite for asserting boundaries in difficult situations.

These exercises are all variations on a theme. Each one is meant to help you lean into your distinctness.

CODEPENDENCY, COUNTERDEPENDENCY, AND ASSERTIVENESS

There's one more aspect of inner boundaries to investigate before we move on to the practice of communicating boundaries to others. I want you to sense whether your personal boundaries tend to be too weak, too rigid, or well-balanced. When setting boundaries, some people are lax while others are inflexible. These two extremes can be respectively characterized by the relational styles of codependency and counterdependency. We'll discuss both, as well as the relational style of assertiveness, which is closer to middle ground.

Codependent individuals tend to have low self-esteem and feel overly responsible for the well-being of others. They tend to form relationships in which they are caretakers for dependent people. Because codependents need to feel needed in order to feel valued, they often attract individuals who are unstable or in need of help. Then they may give beyond their means, ignoring their boundaries and sacrificing themselves until they become frustrated and resentful.

Codependency also has to do with control. To maintain the codependent bond, a codependent person may enable another person to remain dependent on them. Because codependents become easily enmeshed with other people, they often have trouble sensing where their boundaries ought to be. For the same reason, they may have trouble respecting other people's boundaries; they may give unsolicited advice, insert themselves in situations that are none of their business, and tell others what is best for them. Can you relate to this as a healer type, or does this sound like anyone in your life?

In the language of attachment styles, codependency is highly correlated with anxious, insecure attachment. People with an anxious and insecure attachment style tend to bring anxiety to their relationships and require a lot of reassurance and validation. They often have difficulty trusting people, yet they fear being alone.

Addiction often co-occurs with codependency, as the codependent person unintentionally enables the addict to continue their dependence. Coping with loved ones in the throes of addiction requires what's called "loving detachment": refusal to enable addictive behaviors while

HEALER HIGHLIGHT

"My husband was diagnosed with a rare, aggressive blood cancer and died six months after a stem cell transplant. As he was dying, my young adult daughter entered rehab for alcohol abuse and relapsed six times in one year. It was exhausting managing my husband's dying process in parallel with my daughter's near-death experience with alcohol. One month before my husband passed, my son found my daughter vomiting blood. I was hoping to manage one crisis at a time, but my daughter was taken to the ER that day and entered rehab several days later. She was in rehab when her father passed. Becoming active in Al-Anon when my daughter was in rehab and relapsing helped me understand boundaries and avoid enabling her, so that I could support my daughter without draining myself completely."—SUE from New Jersey still expressing care and concern. We must set boundaries and prioritize self-preservation, yet keep the door open should the addict seek help. It's a fine line to walk between enabling and abandoning. Support groups like Al-Anon provide a caring community for the friends and family of addicts. Members learn positive detachment strategies, reclaim inner peace, and determine what they can and cannot control in these complex relationships.

At the opposite extreme of relational styles, we have counterdependency. Counterdependent people often have boundaries that are too strict and rigid. They put up walls to protect themselves and keep others from getting too close, often because they have been hurt or taken advantage of in the past. These are the people who avoid vulnerability, apply strict rules to their relationships, and hold others to irrationally high standards. If a counterdependent person encounters a behavior they don't like in another person, they are apt to cut that person out of their life rather than confront the issue. They also tend to overgeneralize and develop fixed ideas about others. For example, if a counterdependent person asks a friend for help moving and that friend bails at the last minute, the counterdependent person might say, "Of course my friend bailed. People always bail when you really need them. I can't rely on anyone." They are super independent, often believing they don't need anyone because they can do everything on their own. But on the inside, they are usually lonely and lack meaningful connection.

Counterdependency is highly correlated with an avoidant, insecure attachment style. People with an avoidant and insecure attachment style are self-directed and self-contained. They often go out of their way to avoid emotionally charged conversations and situations, as well as commitment and intimacy. They easily feel suffocated when others try to get close to them.

Codependents and counterdependents represent two personality type extremes, and both approaches are unhealthy. It is not ideal to be too self-protective and closed off *or* to be so enmeshed with others that you have no sense of self. In either case, you are depriving yourself of true intimacy with others and avoiding love. Codependents may feel they are unworthy of love, so they settle for being needed. Counterdependents may feel that love is too dangerous, so they settle for being lonely.

The goal is to be somewhere in the middle of these extremes and to choose relationships that are balanced and mutually supportive. People who have an assertive relational style tend to strike this balance. Their personal boundary is more like a semipermeable membrane. They allow some people and some kinds of energy in while keeping others out, as and when they so choose. Setting healthy boundaries means being assertive: able to stand up for yourself without being aggressive or harsh. Assertive people understand that setting boundaries is a form of self-care and that taking care of themselves is the best way to take care of others. They also know that if they hold back from expressing their needs, they will harbor resentment in their relationships, and resentment gets in the way of connection.

An assertive relational style is correlated with a secure attachment style. A secure attachment style develops when someone grows up in an environment where they get consistent attunement from their caretakers and can rely on love being unconditional. This leads to an internalized sense of security that they then bring with them to all their relationships.

If in someone's childhood attunement was erratic, love was given conditionally, or there were disruptions in the caregiving relationship, that sense of internal security doesn't form. People who grow up in those environments typically wind up with a form of insecure attachment: anxious-insecure, where the fear of losing connection leads to codependency, or avoidant-insecure, which involves the fear of being trapped by connection.

Do you see how self-love, self-compassion, and self-awareness help you separate from codependent or counterdependent relational styles and cultivate more assertiveness? We are assertive when we are secure in ourselves. I've often seen people get the advice that to internalize a sense of secure attachment, they need to find a sort of replacement parent—a therapist or romantic partner with whom they can learn how to form a secure attachment. If you've found such a person, that's great. However, an alternative way to become more internally secure is to practice assertive boundary setting.

💚 *Which of these relational styles (codependent, counter-dependent, or assertive) best characterizes you?*

PROTECTING YOUR ENERGY

As healers, we tend to be generous with our time and energy. We want to show up for others and help however we can. But to avoid burnout, we have to be just as generous with ourselves. This means setting boundaries around how, when, and with whom we share our energy.

Start paying attention to which people and situations drain or energize you. Notice when you feel depleted after interacting with certain people. Notice when you feel recharged after spending time alone or with a particular friend who nourishes your soul. Tracking your energy levels throughout your day may reveal a lot about where you need to set firmer boundaries.

If someone in your life is draining your energy, you may need to limit the time you spend interacting with them or set some ground rules around when and how often you are available to talk. You can also practice visualizing an energetic shield around you when interacting with them so their energy doesn't permeate you.

Additionally, make sure you have alone time built into your schedule so you have opportunities to recharge. Take social media breaks and set boundaries around when you are available online as well. Limit volunteering for extra tasks when your plate is already full. Essentially, become very protective of your mental, emotional, physical, and spiritual energy. Treat your energy like the precious resource it is.

♡ *What are your main energy drains? How can you set better boundaries to protect your energy? Make a list of specific people, situations, and commitments you need to set firmer limits with.*

COMMUNICATING WITH KINDNESS

We can't control the way other people react to our boundaries, but we can control the way we communicate them. As Brené Brown puts it, "Clear is kind. Unclear is unkind."[1] So how can we communicate our boundaries clearly and effectively? To help you get the hang of it, here are some example scenarios of what clear and healthy boundaries look like.

Scenario 1: Your close friend is having relationship issues, and she's been calling you for support multiple times per week over the past few months. You can see clearly that she is in an unhealthy relationship, and your conversations have become repetitive and one-sided.

Example boundary: "I'm noticing that we've been having the same conversations about your relationship for a while now, and not much is changing. I care about you and want to support you, but our friendship has started to feel unbalanced. I'd like to take a break from talking about your relationship to see if we can break out of these roles we've gotten into with each other."

Scenario 2: Your mother constantly offers you advice when you just want her to listen.

Example boundary: "I know you have my best interests in mind and want to support me. I would feel more supported if you could listen to me and offer empathy instead of trying to give me advice."

Scenario 3: Your coworker asks if you can help out with a high-priority project, but you're already feeling overwhelmed with the projects you are currently working on.

Example boundary: "I understand this is urgent, but I want to do my best work, and I already have a lot on my plate. I am not able to take on another project right now."

Scenario 4: Your son asks if he can borrow $300 to pay his rent and promises this will be the last time. You have lent him money numerous times already, and he hasn't paid any of it back.

Example boundary: "At this point, I'm no longer willing to support you financially. If there's something else I can do to support you, let me know."

Scenario 5: You are a health coach, and you've been giving a discounted rate to a client for months. Now that the client wants to sign up for another six-month program, you want to increase your rate.

Example boundary: "I want to let you know I've increased my rates since your last program, from $80 to $100 per session. I'd love to continue working together, so I hope that works for you. Let me know and I'll forward you the new paperwork."

You might be formulating a dozen new boundaries you'd like to set in your life as you read this, but I suggest starting slowly. Figure out which boundaries are most urgent, then experiment with setting one boundary at a time. If you are very new to boundary-setting, take the time to evaluate how it feels and how others respond to you. Like any new skill, sometimes you have to be not-so-good at it for a while before you find your groove. For some people, that could mean your language is too careful or meek and therefore not clear enough. For others, you might wind up coming across much harsher than you meant to or acting more entitled than you realized. Both scenarios create another set of problems to deal with! Be willing to take feedback and adjust your approach as you go.

Effective communication truly is an art form. Even though I provided a handful of examples, there's no better way to learn this art than by listening to people who have developed some mastery in it. Two great places to encounter such people are in groups that practice authentic relating[2] and classes that teach nonviolent communication.[3] If you live in a major city, you may be able to find these kinds of groups near you, and they can be found online as well.

♡ *What is one boundary you need to set with someone in your life? What has kept you from setting this boundary up to this point? Write down what communicating this boundary would sound like if you spoke it aloud or sent it in writing. Focus on being clear, concise, and kind.*

DOS AND DON'TS OF
SETTING BOUNDARIES

Here are some dos and don'ts to pay attention to when setting a boundary:

Do

1. *Know your limits and values.* Before you can communicate your boundaries to others, you have to

know what is and isn't acceptable to you. The more self-awareness and self-knowledge you have, the better you will understand your limits and needs. That self-knowledge will make it easier to communicate boundaries with others. Remember, every person is different. Just because one person finds a certain behavior or situation acceptable, doesn't mean you will.

2. *Be direct.* If someone invites you to an event you don't want to attend or asks you to do a favor you don't want to do, don't say "maybe" or "we'll see" if you know your answer is no. When you try to pacify others or let them down gently, you give them false hope and prevent them from making other plans. You also give yourself another job later: saying no closer to the actual task, event, or invitation. So be clear, direct, and as prompt as possible in delivering your answer.

3. *Be concise.* When setting a boundary, saying less is usually better than providing a long explanation. Using too many words can actually make you appear less confident in your boundary, like you are justifying it instead of owning it. Long explanations also give others room to challenge your boundary. Keep it brief—just concisely state what you want, need, and expect.

4. *Say it like a first grader.* Use simple, uncomplicated vocabulary a child could understand. Rather than intellectualizing your feelings, speak plainly and directly. If another person does something to upset you, don't launch into an academic thesis. Instead, you can simply state, "That hurt my feelings. Please don't talk to me that way again."

5. *Focus on solutions, not problems.* The key here is telling the other person what you want, need, or expect. Saying, "I hate it when you invite me to dinner and then show up late," is not a boundary. It's a complaint. To communicate this as a boundary, say, "It makes me feel like you don't value me when you invite me out and then don't show up on time. In the future, can you add in more buffer time and ask me to meet you at a time that is realistic for you?" Focusing on solutions instead of problems minimizes drama.

6. *Align your actions with your words.* If you tell someone you aren't going to tolerate a certain behavior, you need to also say it through your actions. Let's say a friend violates one of your boundaries. What happens then? Are you going to end your friendship? If you set a boundary with a family member that gets violated, are you going to reduce your relationship to email only? Whatever you say the consequence of violating your boundary is going to be, it's important

that you follow through with that consequence. Match your actions to your words by actually doing what you say you're going to do. When you act against the boundaries you set, or set boundaries that are wishy-washy, you give other people the message that they can push you to get what they want. If you want others to respect your boundaries, be consistent and stick to your word.

7. *Make it a policy.* If you are worried another person will take a boundary personally or develop hurt feelings, try this trick from Sarah Knight's book *The Life-Changing Magic of Not Giving a F*ck*: present your boundary as a personal policy.[4] For example, if a coworker adds you to a group text with ten other coworkers and you don't want to be on it, you can say, "I don't do group text messages. It's too distracting for me when my phone vibrates all day long. Feel free to text me separately once everyone figures out a plan." This way, no one feels targeted or singled out.

8. *Address issues as they arise.* The moment you realize someone is violating a boundary, speak up. The longer you allow yourself to stew in negative feelings, the likelier it is that resentment will build and cause you to express your boundary in an unhealthy way.

Don't

1. *Don't wait for other people to figure out what you need.* A common mistake people make when setting boundaries is failing to communicate those boundaries out loud. No one can read your mind, so if you don't communicate your needs clearly, others may not be aware they are overstepping a boundary. Instead of brewing silently in resentment, speak up.

2. *Don't ignore your needs to keep the peace or make other people happy.* Many of us learned from a young age to put the needs of others before our own and to doubt ourselves when negative feelings arise. But anytime your gut is telling you no or you feel violated in any way, it is important to pay attention to that feeling and communicate it if needed. This creates authentic connection, whereas repressing your true feelings only disconnects you from yourself and others.

3. *Don't gossip or complain about others.* For example, if your friend borrows your favorite jacket and doesn't return it, don't complain to everyone you know about it and say nothing to your friend. Instead, confront your friend directly, ask for your jacket back, and explain that moving forward, you don't want her to borrow items of yours unless she can return them within a reasonable amount of time.

4. *Don't offer time, help, money, or other resources you can't afford to share.* Even when they don't have the means to give, healers tend to reflexively say yes when others make requests of them. But that yes is often motivated by guilt or obligation rather than an authentic wish to give. As a rule of thumb, only say yes to requests you are able to fulfill without resentment. Just because you have the means to meet a request, doesn't mean you have to say yes. For example, if your sister asks to borrow money from you, you can say no if saying yes would make you feel resentful, even if you have the funds. If your neighbor asks you to help him move and you have no plans that day other than watching Netflix in your pajamas, you can say no and spend the day doing nothing. You have the right to conserve your time, energy, and resources in whatever ways you wish, even when you have the means to give.

5. *Don't attack another person's character.* When setting boundaries, it's usually best to leave a person's character out of it. An example of attacking another person's character would be to say, "What kind of person knocks on my door without calling first?" Just because someone knocks on your door without checking first, that doesn't make them a bad person. It just means they overstepped a boundary they didn't know

about because you haven't communicated it. If you express your boundary and it happens again, that's a different story. But the first time you communicate a boundary, stick to the behavior that bothered you and what you need or expect moving forward.

6. *Don't make empty threats or give ultimatums you don't plan to follow through with.* There is no need to use threats or scare tactics to coerce others into doing the things you need them to do (e.g., "If you don't come pick up your stuff by the end of today, I'm going to throw it in the garbage"). Instead of making exaggerated threats you don't intend to follow through on, be honest with yourself and others about your boundaries and limits, then align your actions with your words.

7. *Don't try to control other people through your boundaries.* Boundaries are meant to protect you, *not* enable you to control others. For example, you might tell your partner, "I don't want you to go through my phone," and that would be perfectly fair. You are entitled to set boundaries around your personal items. But if you were to say to your partner, "I can't be in a relationship with you unless you let me go through your phone," that's different. That is not a boundary but an attempt to control your partner with an ultimatum. Healthy boundaries do *not* include

manipulating another person to get what you want, trying to manage aspects of another person's life that have nothing to do with you, or demanding that someone think or behave in certain ways.

8. *Don't be afraid to say no.* Not all boundaries require thoughtful language. Sometimes, simply saying no is enough. No need to apologize or overexplain. "No" is a complete sentence. This is especially true in situations where someone is trying to coerce you into doing something personally violating, dangerous, or unlawful. Just say, "No."

♡ *Which of these boundary pointers speak to you? Is there one you want to make sure to remember to try?*

RESPONDING TO PUSHBACK

This is the part where a lot of people get knocked off their horses. They communicate a boundary and use the right language, but then someone reacts poorly, and they start second-guessing themselves. Has this ever happened to you? It is healthy to have standards for yourself and to know how to say no. Setting boundaries does *not* make you mean or selfish. But it can be easy to forget this when faced with pushback and the discomfort of disappointing others.

Unfortunately, even when you make every effort to communicate boundaries with kindness, there will be people who will try to make you feel guilty for needing what you need. Even when people don't like your boundaries, it doesn't mean you are a selfish or rude person for setting them. In healthy relationships, you are able to set boundaries without being made to feel guilty for doing so.

Some common ways people might challenge your boundaries include the following:

- **Ignoring:** They act like they didn't hear your boundary and continue the behavior you've requested they change.

- **Challenging:** They attack your character or challenge what you say you need (e.g., "You're only vegan because it's trendy. Eat a hamburger.").

- **Justifying:** They justify their offending behavior or make excuses as to why they don't need to respect your boundary (e.g., "I had a right to go through your phone because you have lied to me in the past.").

- **Testing:** They continue their offending behavior in a sneaky way so they can continue acting as they like without you noticing (e.g., You tell your roommate you don't want her to smoke cigarettes in the apartment, so she smokes out of her bedroom window when you aren't home).

- **Denying:** They deny their behavior or make you feel irrational for asserting a need (e.g., "I didn't interrupt you. You're being too sensitive.").

- **Guilt-tripping:** They try to make you feel guilty for asserting your boundary in an effort to manipulate you into doing what they want (e.g., You tell your mother you aren't going to fly home for Thanksgiving this year, and she says, "But your father and I are getting older. We may not have that many Thanksgivings left.").

When faced with rejection, it's common to blame ourselves, feeling guilty for having needs or expectations. This guilt stems from being caring, empathetic people who were taught to question our own judgment. But feeling guilty doesn't necessarily mean you did something wrong. Guilt is just part of your programming, and it can be weaponized to make you feel bad for having basic wants and boundaries. It is not your duty to be everything for everyone around you at all times or to regulate other people's emotions. You have a responsibility to nurture and protect yourself first.

On the upside, disappointing others and handling unhealthy reactions to your boundaries gets easier with practice. As a start, rather than questioning yourself in those challenging moments, try tolerating the discomfort instead. Acknowledge your feelings but release the expectation of control. You can't force other people to accept what you're saying or to change, but you can feel proud of yourself for having the courage to communicate your truth. I promise that the more you do this, the more you will let go of the impulse to control what other people feel. You will also start to recognize which relationships in your life might be problematic; whenever someone makes you feel difficult or crazy for wanting to take care of yourself, that's a powerful clue. Your next job becomes navigating how you want to proceed in those relationships.

Often, the people who make you feel bad for standing up for what you need are unhappy themselves. They might try to control you because they lack control over their own lives or the ability to trust themselves and maintain boundaries of their own. It can be especially challenging to assert new boundaries with family members or people you have known for many years, because they may have gotten used to you playing a certain role. So, it can be easy to slip into behaviors that do not serve us simply because they are so well ingrained.

Here are a few ways you might respond when someone challenges a boundary:

- **Restate your boundary** (e.g., "You just made another comment about my weight. I have told you clearly I don't want you to comment about my body.")

- **Give a consequence** (e.g., "If you continue to make comments about my weight, I am not going to visit you anymore.") Remember to state only consequences you are willing to follow through with. Don't make empty threats.

- **Disengage**. Walk away, hang up the phone, and decline future invitations to spend time together.

You have the right to set boundaries in any relationship, even with the most difficult people. You also have the right to let go of relationships with people who do not respect your boundaries. As unnerving as this can be, moving your life into alignment with your authentic truth is the point of doing this work. It isn't your job to convince other people to respect your boundaries. Your job is only to observe how others react to you asserting your boundaries and then decide what you need to do to take care of yourself.

♡ *How are you at dealing with pushback in general? Can you recognize it for what it is? Are you confident in reasserting yourself a second or third time, or could you use more practice?*

SETTING BOUNDARIES FOR YOURSELF

Boundaries for yourself? This might sound like an odd concept, as most of us think of boundaries as limits we set with other people. But being a self-respecting adult also means having boundaries for yourself. If you are able to eat a few cookies and not finish the entire package, or if you go to work every day so you can pay your bills, then you already know what having personal guidelines feels like. Even choosing to go for a run instead of relaxing in bed in the morning is an example of delayed gratification—the opposite of instant gratification. When we practice delayed gratification, we do things that are in our best interest even if they aren't necessarily comfortable in the moment. But most of us have at least one area in our lives where our personal boundaries could use some improvement.

Maybe you're really good at setting limits for yourself when it comes to food, but you have trouble sticking to your financial budget. Or maybe you drink too much coffee, watch too much TV, or spend too much time on social media. Many factors influence why we might find it difficult to set limits for ourselves in certain areas. If there is an area of your life where you've become excessive, it could be a sign that your life is out of balance, or it could be that you grew up with caregivers who didn't model healthy habits or set healthy limits for you. For example, I come from a family of smokers, so I used smoking as a vice when I was young, until I found the will to quit. Take a moment now to think about an area of your life where you struggle to set healthy limits for yourself. What can you trace that back to?

Although our parents and caretakers usually try to do their best, the people who raise us have enormous influence over how good we are at setting boundaries with other people and ourselves. Ideally, parents should set boundaries for their kids that are reasonable—not too harsh and not too lax. When kids learn healthy boundaries from a young age, they come to understand the value of setting limits for themselves as a form of self-care and are able to set healthy personal limits into adulthood.

But if your caretakers set rules for you that were overly strict, you might struggle with self-trust and self-connection. Why? Because your parents didn't give you the space to explore making your own judgments and practice relying on your own instincts to make decisions. You probably also received the message that it was bad or wrong to trust your own instincts. On the other hand, being raised by very lax parents or in an environment lacking rules and structure can also put you at a disadvantage. Kids need structure and consistency to feel safe. They need to know they are contained in some way and that there are people looking out for them. Otherwise, they might struggle with impulse control.

Despite what your upbringing taught you about boundaries, you have the opportunity now as an adult to re-parent your inner child. The first step is examining the areas of your life where you could use more structure. Next, ask yourself, "What decisions would I make for myself if I were a loving, attuned parent?" This should enable you to envision boundaries for yourself that align with your goals and values.

For example, let's say you struggle to set boundaries

with social media. Ask yourself, "If I were my own loving, attuned parent, what would I do to set some boundaries in this area?" You decide you will take a break from all social media for one full week. This means you will delete social media apps from your phone and completely abstain from checking your accounts so you can start filling your time with other activities. Then, after a week, you will limit yourself to thirty minutes of social media per day. You commit to using a timer on your phone to keep yourself accountable. You then decide that every Sunday, you will unplug from technology completely.

Establishing boundaries for yourself, just like establishing boundaries with others, gets easier with practice. The more you practice, the lighter you will feel. When you stop saying yes to people and things that aren't serving you, you will feel more confident and less resentful. You'll open up more space in your life to take care of yourself and experience joy. Just remember to take it one step at a time. Make changes gradually and remember to practice self-compassion. It can also help to have at least one accountability partner, a person you can trust to hold you accountable to the limits you set for yourself.

♡ *When you were growing up, did your caretakers set healthy and reasonable boundaries for you? What is one boundary you need to set for yourself? What has kept you from setting this boundary up to this point?*

Write the boundary down as a note to yourself, and focus on being clear, concise, and kind.

SELF-LOVE CHECKLIST FOR HEALERS

To conclude this chapter, I have put together the following self-love checklist, because setting healthy boundaries and asking for what we need ultimately comes down to loving and valuing ourselves. These items double as affirmations and will be especially helpful if you have a tendency toward people-pleasing, codependency, or counterdependency. Feel free to recite them out loud and refer back to them as often as needed. Remember, it takes repetition to undo the programming that has been consistently instilled in you throughout your life.

- ☐ I am good, even when I am not giving.
- ☐ I openly communicate my feelings, needs, and desires.
- ☐ I accept that it is not my job to fix others nor to solve their problems.
- ☐ I ask for help when I need it.
- ☐ I let others face the consequences of their actions.
- ☐ I respond to calls, texts, and emails when I have the capacity to do so.
- ☐ I choose myself, even when doing so brings feelings of guilt or shame.

☐ I am equipped to tolerate the discomfort of disappointing others.

☐ I hold others accountable for communicating their feelings, needs, and desires.

☐ I set boundaries that protect my mental, emotional, spiritual, and physical well-being.

☐ I release the expectation that I should be perfect.

☐ I surrender to uncertainty and things that are out of my control.

☐ I trust my intuition.

☐ I release, with love and acceptance, relationships, habits, and circumstances that do not serve me.

☐ I open my heart and mind to embrace growth and change.

☐ I deserve to receive the type of care I put out into the world.

☐ I am worthy of being loved.

☐ I do not owe anyone anything.

☐ I am enough.

PART IV

HEAL THE HEALER TOOL KIT

CHAPTER 9

NAME WHAT YOU AUTHENTICALLY VALUE

───────── ♡ ─────────

I N THE PREVIOUS SEVERAL CHAPTERS, WE focused on recovering from trauma—essentially, healing from the past. Next, we'll focus on ongoing growth. Discovering which inner resources you didn't develop when you were young and strengthening them now will help you become more resilient for the future.

Think of these final chapters as your tool kit for healing the healer: a set of skills and resources that will allow you to emerge stronger from the challenges of the healing role and to protect yourself against future burnout. To set the foundation for making use of this tool kit, we need to start out by clarifying our values.

As human beings, we have an innate need to be authentic—to be in touch with our needs and desires and to share our truth with others. But as we move through life, we learn to follow rules, do what is expected of us, and ignore many of our natural instincts. Many of us grew up with parents who didn't always hold space for us to express our feelings. Maybe they lacked the emotional skills or ability to attune to us, so we learned to bury our emotions and suppress aspects of our true nature.

After many years of this kind of self-denial, we lose self-connection and self-trust. We get so caught up in what we should be doing to please the people around us that we stop paying attention to our own needs or simply choose not to express them. Instead, we become "nice" and congenial. We turn away from the authentic truth that lives within us because it feels dangerous, and because we are afraid of judgment, ridicule, and not belonging.

Then we wake up one day and wonder why we aren't happy. The thing is, even when we push down our truth and do a really great job of acting like we're okay on the outside, in our heart and soul, we never forget who we truly are. Our bodies hold the wisdom of our past and our most authentic desires for the future. If you relate to any of what I am saying here, then you know the feeling. When you aren't doing what you are meant to be doing with your life, or living where you want to be living, or loving who you want to be loving, you feel a sense of shame and despair. Maybe you even lose touch with reality. This sense of self-betrayal is there whether you choose to tune in to it or not.

This inner knowing is there for a reason: to guide you to the path you are meant to be on. But many of us ignore it, at least until something life-altering happens to jolt us awake, like a near-death experience or getting diagnosed with a serious illness. When you hear that little voice of truth inside, it's important to listen because it will find a way to get through to you, one way or another. To connect intimately with others, we need to step out of the roles we have been taught to play and allow ourselves to be truly seen.

VALUES IN THE MODERN WORLD

As of 2022, Internet users worldwide spent an average of two and a half hours per day on social media.[1] This is amazing to me when I consider that a few decades ago, hardly anyone even owned a computer. Social media and smartphones only came about in the early 2000s, becoming more mainstream in the 2010s. Today, we are exposed to a never-ending stream of marketers and influencers competing for our time and attention. It is more important than ever to have a mind of your own as we are faced daily with people who are literally paid to influence our thinking. If we don't have grounded core values in the modern world, we're likely to be wishy-washy and all over the place. Whatever is trending on social media is going to become our life.

For example, glute workouts have become a fitness obsession for women in recent years, mostly because of the Kardashians. You can go to pretty much any gym in the country and see women doing all kinds of exercises to grow and shape their glutes. If you wish to have a healthy, fit body, there's certainly nothing wrong with having strong glute muscles. But many women trying to achieve this aesthetic are following a trend, spending disproportionately more time working their glutes than any other muscle group. They are being influenced by a beauty standard that wasn't mainstream a few years ago.

Modern culture prompts us to navigate the world based on what is trending at the moment rather than what is integral to us as individuals. This is why it is necessary to ask yourself, "Who am I? What is important to *me*? What is my basic belief system? What are my non-negotiables?" and, most importantly, "Do I love myself as I am right now?" With the cyclone of trends swirling around us, it's easy for people to confuse more likes with more love and miss the concept of genuine self-love. It's hard not to fall into the trap of thinking, "Maybe I will finally love myself if I get fitter or get more followers on social media." But knowing and loving ourselves at the core level requires us to stop scrolling and focus our attention inward.

CONNECTING TO YOUR VALUES

When we are disconnected from our values, it's like walking around blindfolded. It is difficult to set goals and make decisions if you have no sense of what matters to you. When we are connected to our values, they serve as a compass, guiding us where we need to go. So, how do we attune to ourselves though all the noise and influences around us? How can we reconnect with the voice within us that knows what we want and need in order to be happy?

One way to connect with your values is by slowing down and silencing your mind. For many of us, the COVID-19 pandemic forced us to re-evaluate our lives and what is truly important to us. This major world event served as a wake-up call. It reminded us that life as we know it can change in an instant and nothing is guaranteed. But now that we are no longer living in lockdown, many of us have gotten lost again in the distractions of our fast-paced world. Again, we are living on autopilot, going through the motions from one day to the next.

We need to relearn how to be intentional, slow, and present, whether we are in crisis mode or not. Hit the pause button as often as you need to, and go someplace where you can escape the noise of the world around you. Reflect on what matters to you and how your life needs to look to align with those values. Mindfulness and self-connection are key throughout this process.

To stay connected to your values even as they evolve, it's helpful to have a daily practice, like meditation or journaling, that guides your attention toward your internal experience.

AUTHENTIC VALUES VERSUS LIMITING BELIEFS

As we connect with what matters to us, we need to discern between values that are genuinely important to us personally and those that were instilled in us by other people. One way to tell the difference is to examine the personal stories that are connected to your values. Ask yourself, "Did this value arise out of something deep and authentic in me in response to this situation, or did it get imprinted on me by someone else, who may have been living in fear or denial? Did another person or group force me to believe this because it served *them*, or because they didn't have the skills to attune to me and my needs?"

For example, let's say you value generosity, and I ask you, "Why? Can you share an experience that comes to mind when you think of generosity?" You recall a time as a young adult when your credit card got declined at the grocery store, and the stranger behind you swiped her card to pay for your groceries. This sounds like an authentic value that developed out of feeling cared for by a generous stranger. Or maybe you value assertiveness, which ties back to a time when you stood up to your childhood bully and finally got him to leave you alone. This also sounds like an authentic value, born out of a moment of courage.

On the other hand, let's say you value keeping a perfectly clean house that's always well organized. You trace this back to a story about how your mother always kept an immaculately clean house and made you feel guilty anytime you made any sort of mess as a child. When you think about having a messy home, it fills you with a sense of anxiety and dread. Well, it sounds like you developed this so-called value because you wanted to keep your mom happy and avoid being punished. So this one sounds more like a limiting belief. In this case, your mother may have been obsessive about cleaning because of her own shortcomings or fear of not being in control. Her anxiety then got passed on to you.

Do you see the difference? Of course, this explanation of how values develop is a bit oversimplified. What we come to value is the product of many experiences and influences. But as you practice connecting your values to personal stories, you will start to feel the difference between authentic values and limiting beliefs. When a value is authentic, it arises out of a certain part of your body. It is a totally unique sensation. A personal story connected to an authentic value might fill your heart with joy and gratitude, or it might empower you, connecting you to your inner resilience. Any values that connect to experiences where you were courageous or followed your heart and did the right thing despite what others thought are probably authentic. Any "values" that make you feel stressed or weighted down are probably limiting beliefs.

Something else you could do to help you discern between authentic values and limiting beliefs is to create a values word web. Let's say you value community service. On a blank sheet of paper, write *community service* in the middle of the page and circle it. Then draw a line out of that center circle and write down another word, phrase, or example that connects to community service for you, e.g., *volunteering at the soup kitchen in high school*, and circle it. If your dad signed you up for that specific volunteering opportunity, you might draw another line branching off from that circle that says *Dad*. And so on.

If you continue this exercise, drawing more branches out from your center circle, you will likely find that your values connect back to many different people and experiences. When you are able to view the full picture of where a particular value originates from, you should gain a clearer sense of whether or not that value is authentic for you.

LIVING ACCORDING TO YOUR VALUES

Living according to your values involves taking risks and trusting your truth, even when it goes against what others expect of you. This may be uncomfortable, but it almost always pays off. When you are clear about what lights a fire within you, you become empowered to take action. You start relying on your values to guide you instead of being guided by other people's limitations. And you get to design your future according to what matters most to you.

As you continue to clarify and solidify your values, remember that what makes one person happy is not necessarily going to make another person happy. We all have different life purposes, interests, and things that bring us joy. It's up to you to decide what fulfillment and freedom look like for you. After that, you can surround yourself with others who share similar values.

Complete the following prompts to help increase your awareness around what you value in different areas of your life. Take your time with each question, noticing what comes up and meditating on your answer if you need to. But don't overthink it; trust your instincts and try to answer each question with your heart. When you are done, you can assess which areas of your life are in alignment with your values and which are not.

1. List what you value most when it comes to:
   - **Family** (e.g., openness, respecting boundaries)

- **Friendships** (e.g., similar interests, meaningful conversations)
- **Intimate partnerships** (e.g., loyalty, quality time)
- **Career** (e.g., job security, flexible schedule)
- **Where you live** (e.g., near the ocean, good school district)
- **Money** (e.g., being able to afford travel, long-term investments)
- **Physical activity** (e.g., group fitness, being outdoors)
- **Your home environment** (e.g., organized, cozy)
- **How you spend your free time** (e.g., freedom, serenity)

2. What is not important to you? List some things that other people seem to value that you value less or not at all (e.g., holiday traditions, sports, having the newest iPhone). You may use the same categories from step 1 to guide your thinking.

3. Name a few people in your life who share your values. How does being around these people make you feel?

4. Name a few people in your life who *do not* share your values. How does being around these people make you feel?

5. What would your life look like if you decided to live 100 percent according to your values? How about if

you weren't concerned with fitting in or disappointing others?

6. How would living according to your values impact your future?

WHAT TO LET GO OF

We've talked about overcoming limiting beliefs so you can persevere in life and rise to your true potential. But living according to what you value also requires knowing when to quit: knowing and trusting yourself enough to let go of the things that aren't helping you grow. As you shift, it is only natural that your relationships and commitments will shift, too. And that's okay. To live a less encumbered life, you are going to need to release the things that drain your energy and don't align with your goals and values. When you release the things in your life that aren't serving you, you will feel less resentful, overwhelmed, frustrated, and tired. And you will gain back the energy to create the life you desire.

As you begin to re-evaluate the relationships and commitments in your life, you might need to adjust your expectations or involvement, which can bring up a sense of grief. This is normal. Sometimes, we need to mourn the things we cannot change or the time and energy we sacrificed fighting for things that didn't pan out as we hoped. Giving yourself permission to grieve your disappointments, mistakes, and/or limitations is a form of acceptance. It allows you to eventually move on.

What do you need to change or let go of to create your ideal life? What boundaries do you need to set to protect your vision of ultimate well-being?

Use the following question prompts to start identifying the things you need to release to create a life that supports your values and well-being. These questions are organized into different areas so that you can focus on one important topic at a time. Feel free to skip any areas that do not apply.

Relationships

Are you always the one helping others and never the one receiving support? List any relationships in your life that feel stressful, one-sided, or draining. These can be relationships with friends, family members, coworkers, romantic partners, or other people you interact with regularly.

Of the relationships you wrote down, reflect on which ones you may need to re-evaluate or adjust your involvement in. This doesn't necessarily mean ending the relationships but considering where stronger boundaries or reduced contact may be beneficial. Circle the relationships you want to preserve but with healthier boundaries in place. What specific boundaries or changes to your role do you need to implement in order to make those relationships healthier?

Codependent Behaviors

Do you find yourself overfunctioning in relationships? Do you try to rescue others rather than allowing them to take responsibility for themselves? Do you offer unsolicited advice or take responsibility for other people's emotions? List any codependent behaviors you are willing to let go of.

Counterdependent Behaviors

Do you find yourself putting up walls between yourself and others? Do you resist trusting other people or letting them in for fear of being disappointed? List any counterdependent behaviors you are willing to let go of.

Perfectionist Tendencies

Are you unreasonably hard on yourself and afraid of making mistakes? Do you give 110 percent of yourself to every task, even when perfection isn't required? If you identify as a perfectionist, list any perfectionist tendencies you are willing to release (e.g., "My house doesn't have to be spotless all the time" or "I don't need to put on makeup before going to the gym").

Financial Habits

Have you loaned money to anyone who hasn't paid you back? Have you been overspending and need to implement some financial boundaries for yourself? List any unhealthy financial habits you are ready to let go of.

Health Habits

Are you engaging in any habits that are negatively affecting your physical health (e.g., smoking cigarettes, consuming too much processed food or sugar, sitting too much)? List any harmful health habits you are willing to quit or change.

Work/School

If you work for an employer, do you frequently take on work that is outside the scope of your job title or work extra hours without pay? If you work for yourself, do you undercharge clients for your work and time? Do you fail to take vacations and time off? List any habits around work or school that you are willing to change.

Social Expectations

Have you been following traditions or living according to systems that don't align with your values? How about other people's rules or ideas of happiness and success? List any social expectations you want to stop conforming to.

Social Media

Do you have any habits around social media that you would like to change, such as how much time you spend scrolling each day? Are there any social media accounts you are willing to mute or unfollow because of how they make you feel? List the changes you want to make when it comes to the way you engage with social media.

Chores and Responsibilities

What tasks do you do on a daily or weekly basis that you hate doing?

Would it be possible to let go of any of these tasks? Put an X through any tasks you are willing to let go of entirely.

Of the tasks you need to keep, would it be possible to outsource any of them? Circle any tasks you might be able to outsource to a professional or delegate to someone else.

Anything Else?

Consider other things in your life that may be causing you unnecessary stress or discomfort. List anything you might need to let go of to live according to your values.

Once you start weeding out some of the relationships, habits, and responsibilities that have been crowding your life, you might feel a void. This is completely natural. You were used to all your time being accounted for and not having the bandwidth to consider yourself. When you are preoccupied with other people's needs, you get to avoid addressing your own trauma, grief, and pain. You also get to avoid pursuing your goals and dreams, which is comfortable in the sense that you cannot fail if you don't take any risks. When you open up some space in your life, you are forced to ask yourself, "What now? What do *I* want and need?" That can be scary, especially if you have never asked yourself these questions before.

Having a plan is a good way to lessen some of the inevitable fear of facing this new void. For every hour of your life you reclaim for yourself, what will you spend it on? For every relationship you let go of, can you cultivate a new relationship in its place? Or can you strengthen an existing relationship with someone you like and feel supported by? In the next two chapters, I'll help you identify what to cultivate to transform your current life into one where you feel supported.

OUTSOURCING AND RESOURCE SHARING

Not everyone has money to spare. As you progress in your career as a healer or wellness worker, however, you may find that time becomes a scarcer resource than money. If that's true for you, you might consider outsourcing—hiring others to do the tasks you don't have the time or energy to do yourself. Some of these may be day-to-day tasks, like using the Instacart app to have your groceries delivered to you. Many grocery stores offer similar services. If you need help running errands or taking care of things around the house, Thumbtack and TaskRabbit have online directories you can use to easily hire local taskers. If you're an entrepreneur looking for a freelancer to help with certain aspects of running your business, Upwork and Fiverr are great resources. You can hire professionals to help you create a website, write newsletter copy, design graphics, create a social media ad campaign, and much more.

If you've always done everything yourself, it will probably feel strange to outsource your work to others. Don't let the awkwardness stop you. Allowing other people to do things for you frees you up to focus on your unique contributions.

If paying others to free up your time is not an option for you, sharing resources with people in your personal network may be a workable alternative. In more traditional societies, and in many parts of the world today, people live in close-knit communities where it's easy to help one another with daily tasks. If you're a part of a more individualistic culture and living some distance away from friends and family, sharing resources requires a more deliberate effort. It's worth putting in the energy up front, however, to strengthen your network of mutual support. For instance, you might have a tech-savvy nephew who can help you create a website. Maybe you and a neighbor could take turns cooking meals for each other or taking care of each other's kids. Finding ways to barter, share skills, and trade responsibilities doesn't just lighten your load—it's also a great way to build community.

As we gain the self-knowledge and courage to live more authentically, release what doesn't serve us, and rely more on others, we free up a wealth of time and energy, especially emotional energy. Having more control over where our energy is going means that instead of being drained by the end of each day, we have more to give to ourselves. We develop greater self-connection, self-trust, and self-confidence. We also become better equipped to protect ourselves against future burnout. This is especially important for healers who have a tendency toward operating on autopilot, from a place of disempowerment, and forgetting themselves. When we are truly plugged into ourselves and everything we do, our lives begin to feel simpler and more joyful. We are more present, energized, and optimistic. We operate in a state of flow.

CHAPTER 10

CALL IN YOUR RESOURCES

♡

NOW THAT YOU HAVE MORE CLARITY ABOUT what you value and what you need to release to create the life you desire, it's time to look at what you need to nurture. Given the demanding nature of our work as healers, we can easily get out of balance. It is crucial for us to sustain relationships and practices that recenter and revitalize us.

As a first step, I'm going to ask you to assess how you are currently doing in some important areas: bodywork, physical activity, mindfulness, purpose and meaning, joy and play, rest, sleep, financial self-care, mutually supportive relationships, environment, and sex and physical touch. Later, I'll help you visualize and plan your next steps in these areas. But first, let's get clear about your current relationship with each.

For every area that follows, I've included a brief description, as well as questions meant to focus your awareness on what you are currently doing to prevent burnout and take care of yourself. Write your answers down and keep them handy, because we'll refer back to them in the next chapter. For now, just observe any obvious patterns (such as which areas you're solid in and which areas could use improvement). And keep in mind that an integrative approach to healing means bringing together a variety of different therapies, techniques, and self-care practices in order to nurture and restore balance to all aspects of *you*.

BODYWORK AND OTHER MODALITIES

Bodywork and energy healing encompass a range of hands-on, energy-based therapeutic techniques aimed at rebalancing the body holistically. Examples of bodywork modalities include massage, craniosacral therapy, myofascial release, reflexology, Rolfing, and chiropractic adjustments. These practices use touch to address musculoskeletal issues, release fascial restrictions, stimulate pressure points, and realign the body structurally.

Energy-based modalities like Reiki, healing touch therapy, acupuncture, and Qigong focus on clearing blockages and restoring flow throughout the body's energy system.

Practitioners use light touch or work with the energy field surrounding the skin. The intention is to activate the self-healing abilities of the recipient's body and mind. Sessions occur in calm settings free of stress to establish an environment where recipients feel safe to fully relax into the experience.

HEALER HIGHLIGHT

"I discovered Qigong, an ancient Chinese practice combining breathwork, gentle movements, and meditation in 2011, after years of failing to heal a torn shoulder ligament through Western methods. At thirty, I traveled to China to intensively study Qigong, and I returned home pain-free with my shoulder healed. As a Qigong practitioner, I've been teaching in my community since 2017 and seeing students transform as they deeply reconnect with their bodies. Though my classes are small, it's beautiful to watch Qigong flourish in others as it did for me. I continue practicing daily because Qigong is my medicine—when I don't do it, I feel it. I've learned to live in flow with energy and listen to my body's needs. The beauty of Qigong is that it can be done anywhere. The more I connect with surrounding energy, the more my own qi is strengthened."—**ANGIE** from Australia

Other mind-body practices, such as hypnotherapy, guided imagery, and eye movement desensitization and reprocessing (EMDR), incorporate cognitive, emotional, and somatic processing to address trauma, negative thought patterns, and limiting beliefs held in the body and psyche. Emotional Freedom Technique (EFT), also known as tapping, involves tapping on energy meridian points while mentally focusing on the pain you want to address, restoring balance in the body's energy system.[1]

Newer healing modalities include cold exposure, red light therapy, and infrared saunas. Cold exposure, such as ice baths or cryotherapy, activates the body's natural anti-inflammatory response and stimulates the immune system while increasing metabolism, potentially alleviating pain, improving sleep, and encouraging weight loss.[2] Red light therapy delivers wavelengths that may stimulate cellular energy, reduce inflammation, and improve skin health.[3] Infrared saunas induce detoxifying sweat while surrounding you in healing heat. This improves blood circulation, speeds up muscle recovery, and may decrease depression, anxiety, and stress.[4]

♡ *Do you currently incorporate bodywork or any other therapeutic healing modalities as part of your self-care routine?*

PHYSICAL ACTIVITY

When you're stressed, your body releases hormones such as adrenaline and cortisol. Whether you're being chased by a big dog or stuck in traffic, the body can't tell the difference between a real threat and a perceived one. Either way, you'll be stuck in fight-or-flight mode, meaning your body is physiologically ready to fight or flee. The stress response cycle can't complete itself without physical movement, even after the threat passes. Your body stays tense and physiologically primed for action.

Physical activity works to discharge those built-up stress hormones. It signals to your nervous system that you are safe, so you can relax. Activities like walking, running, dancing, swimming, biking, and weight lifting shift your physiology out of overdrive. This completes the stress cycle and brings your body back to baseline. Plus, it releases feel-good endorphins and serotonin.

In addition to traditional exercise, movement-based healing modalities like yoga, conscious dance, and Tension and Trauma Releasing Exercises (TRE) focus on guiding the body through repetitive motions that promote relaxation.

Yoga coordinates movement with breath to ground the body and calm the nervous system. Studies show yoga can reduce stress, ease anxiety, and improve mood.[5] Conscious or ecstatic dance uses free-form movement to release emotions and shift energy.[6] TRE uses gentle exercises, like shaking, to discharge pent-up stress and tension from the muscles and fascia.[7] Adding these practices to your self-care routine should allow your body to enter a more parasympathetic state.

💚 *How much physical activity do you currently incorporate into your life?*

MINDFULNESS

I highlighted the importance of mindfulness in an earlier chapter as a key factor in developing resilience. Because mindfulness is such an essential resource, I want to bring it back here and talk about some other aspects of it.

Take fifteen seconds to close your eyes and focus on your breathing, then come back. Whenever I do this, it's like, "Whoa! Where am I?" In an instant, I become far more aware of the different sensations in my body and sounds around me. What did you notice? Maybe you felt the saliva in your mouth. Or maybe you noticed a tight muscle in your body, or a sound coming from outside the window. You just practiced mindfulness. See how easy that was?

If you observe the universe in all its vastness, it's like a huge vacuum of stillness. This profound sense of peace in nature reflects the meditative state we're trying to get to—our original way of being. Yet as humans, we often speed along on the bullet train of life, rushing from one thing to the next without stopping to breathe. In doing so, it's easy to lose connection with our deepest truths. Mindfulness practices help interrupt the momentum of daily demands. They act as brakes to decelerate the "bullet train" so we can realign with stillness once more. Some mindfulness practices include the following.

Meditation

A lot of people get heroic and try to meditate for twenty minutes a day or more. They think they need to light a candle and sit on a fancy pillow with their legs crossed a certain way. But meditation is accessible no matter where you are, and you don't have to meditate for twenty minutes to experience the benefits. You can meditate for five minutes a day, or one minute a day, and still enter that space of expanded awareness that comes with bringing attention to your breath, body, and mind.

Breathing Techniques

If you're struggling with stress and anxiety, you can try various breathing exercises to calm your nervous system and relax your body. Begin with just a few minutes a day and increase your time as the exercises become easier. Some common techniques include pursed-lip breathing, diaphragmatic breathing, and alternate nostril breathing. More advanced breathwork techniques, such as holotropic breathwork (HB), can induce altered states of consciousness that may provide healing benefits. Work with a trained facilitator if interested in exploring intense breathwork practices.

Journaling

Writing can have tremendous therapeutic benefits, allowing you to slow down your thoughts and feelings and bring awareness to them. Try journaling for ten minutes daily or for fifteen to twenty minutes a few times a week. You can also try writing Morning Pages, made popular by Julia Cameron in *The Artist's Way*: sit down first thing in the morning and write three pages before you do anything else, allowing your stream of consciousness to flow.

Gratitude Practices

Cultivating gratitude helps to shift your perspective and bring your awareness to the blessings already present in your life. Try writing down three to five things you're grateful for each day. You can also incorporate gratitude reflections into your mindfulness routine.

Grounding in Nature

To de-stress, try going for mindful walks in nature while paying close attention to sights, sounds, and sensations. For some extra grounding, try walking barefoot on grass (sometimes called Earthing), which has a number of health benefits including reducing inflammation and helping the nervous system shift into a parasympathetic state.

Mindful Eating

You can practice mindfulness while you eat by enjoying at least one meal per day with no technology or distractions. Focus on chewing your food slowly, and give awareness to the texture, flavor, and temperature of the food in your mouth. You can even set the mood before a meal by lighting candles, putting on soft music, and creating an ambiance of relaxation.

As a healer, making time for mindfulness is crucial. After absorbing others' energies, mindfulness helps you reset, ground yourself, and trust in the bigger picture. I often say that whatever makes the day turn to night and the night turn to day—what makes the seasons change and keeps all the planets in perfect orbit—can certainly take care of little old me. Whether you call it God, the universe, or a higher power, there is an intelligent rhythm we can tune in to. By practicing mindfulness and letting go of control, we enter the here and now. Even just a minute or two of tuning in to your breathing and senses can realign you with the peaceful stillness beneath life's constant motion. Over time, these practices help balance out our tendency to feel restless and anxious.

♡ *How do you practice mindfulness in your life?*

PURPOSE AND MEANING

Have you ever stopped to wonder why we are all living on this rock called Earth in a huge and infinite universe? So many of us bulldoze through our days with self-importance, preoccupied with our personal problems. But our health improves and our lives become richer when we have a sense of purpose and meaning—when we are able to answer the question, "What is it all for?"

Our sense of purpose and meaning becomes our North Star, giving our lives direction. It motivates us to work toward goals that fulfill us, and it helps us cope when we face life's challenges. All the menial tasks we have to get done every day can feel pretty pointless unless we are connected to something larger. Many people find meaning through doing things that connect them to others. We also find meaning through spirituality, religion, connecting with nature, and going after goals that will leave a positive legacy.

As healers, we feel an innate yearning to help other people. But this task can feel intimidating because of how many people in the world need help. Where do we start? Howard Thurman said, "Do not ask what the world needs. Ask what makes you come alive and go do that, because what the world needs is people who have come alive."[10] Following this advice, it's important to tune in to your intuition and ask yourself questions like, "What activities do I enjoy so much that I lose track of time?"

It's important to note that your purpose doesn't need to be groundbreaking or world-changing. It may be as simple as enjoying your time on earth, growing as a person, or healing your own generational trauma. You don't have to save every suffering person you meet, even if you're a healer. You don't have to always be helping, doing, and contributing to the world.

♡ *Do you feel like you have a sense of purpose and meaning in your life? If not, what do you think might be in the way of that?*

JOY AND PLAY

As healers, we're so focused on helping others that we may forget to allow ourselves to enjoy life. I get it. When you're mired in a to-do list that is never ending, doing anything that isn't productive can feel like a waste of time or add to your stress. But making time to enjoy life's simple pleasures is incredibly important.

American culture teaches us we need to work constantly and live a fast-paced lifestyle if we want to amount to anything. But studies have shown that when we're laughing and having fun, we are healthier and less stressed.[11] Sometimes just enjoying something for the sake of enjoying something, without a specific goal or plan in mind, is the best medicine.

When was the last time you played a board game with friends or family, danced to music in your living room, visited a museum, or did something just for the fun of it?

I remember working with a student who complained once that she couldn't stop playing games on her phone. She called it procrastinating, but I offered the possibility that it was her brain trying to go offline for a while and take a break so it could recharge itself. The guilt this woman felt over playing games on her phone is what made it a problem. It would have been better for her to simply allow herself to play the games, or do something else that would allow her mind to drift and have fun. Sometimes feeling stuck is a sign that we need to take a break and play on purpose.

💙 *What do joy and play look like for you? Do you make time for joy and play in your life?*

REST

Rest means giving your body, mind, and emotions a break. We often think of rest as just physical—lying down when our bodies get tired. But physical rest isn't the only kind of rest we need. We also need mental and emotional rest. Our minds aren't meant to be productive every waking hour, constantly processing information. Sometimes our minds need to go offline. Just like how we need to reboot our computers from time to time, we need to reset our own mental operating systems. And with constant busyness, anxiety, and stress, our nervous systems need rest, too.

Resting can look like napping, reading, listening to soothing music, taking a bath—activities that allow the body and mind to recharge. With rest we become more productive, creative, compassionate, happy, and healthy.

Many of us resist rest as a result of being brainwashed by grind culture. We don't want other people to see us as lazy or unambitious. But resisting rest backfires because our bodies always send us the message to slow down in one way or another. As Tricia Hersey writes in *Rest Is Resistance,* "We must believe we are worthy of rest. We don't have to earn it. It is our birthright. It is one of our most ancient and primal needs."

Rest allows us to reconnect with our bodies, restoring our energy, attention, focus, and motivation. It also allows us to create, dream, wander, and experiment—all vital human experiences. Our bodies need even more rest when we are going through stressful life events and personal struggles. Introverts and highly sensitive people also require more rest and alone time.

♡ *Are you resting your body, brain, and nervous system enough? How much rest do you need in a typical day? What are your favorite ways to rest and recharge?*

SLEEP

Sleep is essential for just about every organ and bodily function. When you sleep, your sympathetic nervous system finally gets a chance to rest. Your brain processes the day's information while your body fights inflammation and repairs damaged tissues, blood vessels, and cells. Getting enough sleep makes us more energized, creative, and alert. It allows us to process, integrate, and retain information, and also helps regulate our weight and hormones.

Chronic sleep deprivation can impair brain functioning, decision-making, focus, and creativity.[12] It can also contribute to chronic health problems like heart disease, kidney disease, high blood pressure, obesity, stroke, diabetes, and depression.[13] When you are sleep deprived, you are unable to operate at your full potential. Because healing work is particularly demanding and emotionally taxing, many healers struggle with sleep issues.

HEALER HIGHLIGHT

"As a therapist who works primarily with victims of sexual assault, I used to struggle with racing thoughts before bed that made sleeping a challenge. I've since realized it is vitally important that I take the time at the end of every workday to decompress and allow my mind to wander and to process the information I've taken in during the day. It also helps me to make physical activity a part of my daily routine, so I can move stress and emotions out of my body."—CHLOÉ from Canada

---

Here are some ways to improve sleep hygiene for healers who have trouble winding down:

- Maintain a regular sleep schedule as much as possible, even on days off. Going to bed and waking up at consistent times reinforces the body's circadian rhythms.

- Power down technology at least thirty minutes before bedtime. Screens emit blue light that disrupts melatonin production. Try reading a book or meditating instead of watching TV or scrolling on your phone.

- Write down racing thoughts to get them out of your head and prevent ruminating in bed.

- Take a warm bath or soak your feet in warm water and Epsom salt to promote relaxation.

- Diffuse calming essential oils like lavender in your bedroom.

- Take magnesium supplements or drink herbal tea before bed.

- Use blackout curtains to make sure your room is dark enough for quality sleep.

- Use a sound machine or listen to soothing music or white noise.

- Give yourself some down time to unwind from your day; avoid working right before bed.

The key is having a wind-down routine to transition out of stress mode so you can relax and get the restorative rest you require.

♥ *Do you typically get enough sleep? Is it usually high or low quality?*

FINANCIAL SELF-CARE

Healers often undervalue themselves financially. Many wellness workers struggle with having the money conversation with potential clients, asking for fair pay, and raising their rates. I have also seen a lot of IIN health coaches give away their services for free because they care deeply about the work they do and want to avoid being "salesy." However, in our commerce-driven society, money is necessary to care for ourselves and others. While not the root of happiness, financial security provides peace of mind that is essential for solving problems. With more income, we also become able to hire other people to support us, which can relieve burnout.

In chapter 5, I talked about how the healer hierarchy undervalues caring work, so by valuing ourselves and our services appropriately, we can spur societal change. Charging fair rates elevates the value of healing roles as perceived by society. As healers, we must embrace financial self-care to sustain ourselves, help others, and shift mindsets around the importance of our work.

HEALER HIGHLIGHT

"I have always felt a deep calling, along with a natural ability, to support others in their healing processes. Although I am trained as a health coach and Reiki Master, I've always viewed healing as a deeply intuitive practice guided more by inner wisdom than formal training. So, I've struggled with the idea of attaching a price to my innate abilities, as I believe healing should flow from genuine intention rather than expectation."—BETH from Ohio

Owning your worth when it comes to your finances—asking for what you deserve, creating a financial plan for yourself, and allowing yourself to flourish in this area—will help you attract more abundance and prosperity in other areas of your life.

♥ *How are you doing with your finances? If you are currently working, do you feel you are being adequately compensated for the work you are doing?*

MUTUALLY SUPPORTIVE RELATIONSHIPS

When I was growing up, I often heard my mother complain about friends or neighbors who didn't return favors. "I've done so much for these people, and they couldn't do this one thing for me," she would say. Because my mom and dad were so generous with their time and resources, they noticed when others didn't reciprocate. As I got older, I found myself having similar gripes. I'd show up for others like it was part of my DNA, but when I needed something in return, those same people wouldn't be there for me.

Our social environment and the individuals we regularly engage with have a significant influence on our emotional well-being. This is especially true for people who are highly empathic. The moods and personalities of the people around us—our family members, coworkers, spouse, and others—are contagious. So, as healers, we need to pay special attention to the quality of our relationships, as many of us tend toward one-sided relationships where we give more than we receive. Are you the friend people call when they need advice? Do you do 80 percent of the listening in most of your relationships while the other person does 80 percent of the talking? Because healers like to feel needed, we are often the caretakers in our families, friendships, and romantic partnerships. As a result, we may feel lonely, isolated, and/or resentful. These feelings then lead us to withdraw socially and isolate ourselves, which is an issue because connecting with others is essential to our health and well-being.

Although we are nourished to some extent through acts of giving, we also need people in our lives who are attuned to us: people who can support, validate, and hold space for us; people who will turn toward our difficult feelings with kindness and compassion; and people who care about our well-being as much as we care about theirs. Receiving emotional support from others helps us process and release our emotions. It can also lower our stress and anxiety levels and increase our sense of purpose and meaning in life. To feel whole, we need to give *and* receive.

Mutually supportive relationships are based on mutual trust, respect, safety, authenticity, compassion, vulnerability, and emotional maturity. Emotionally mature relational partners are responsible, reliable, and considerate of one another. They communicate their needs and respect boundaries. They reciprocate effort, compromise on important issues, and allow one another to be who they authentically are. In chapter 13, I'll talk about the power of community, which takes mutually supportive relationships to the collective level.

♡ *Who do you share mutually supportive relationships with in your life? How would you describe those relationships? In what ways do you support one another?*

ENVIRONMENT

Thirty years ago, I moved to New York City to start the Institute of Integrative Nutrition, because New York City feels like the center of the universe. There is so much happening there. But for the first few years, I couldn't afford rent, so I was sleeping on a couch in the office of the school. I was also using that office to see health coaching clients during the day. After several sessions, I would take a break and step out into the staircase to smoke a cigarette. I had a whole routine—take a few puffs and then go to the bathroom, wash my face, and gargle so I wouldn't smell like smoke when I met my next client. In many ways, I felt like a fraud. Here I was coaching others on how to eat better and improve their well-being, but I couldn't make it through a day without cigarettes.

I knew I needed to change, so I took a bus up to Kripalu, a yoga retreat center in Massachusetts. I continued to visit Kripalu once a month. Sometimes I paid to stay there, but I also figured out how to stay for free by sleeping on the floor in the library. At Kripalu, life was much slower. It felt soothing to be surrounded by nature after all the time I spent in a concrete jungle. At some point while at Kripalu, I noticed that whenever I was there, I didn't crave cigarettes. This helped me realize how much the stress of the city was affecting me.

When Kripalu started experiencing financial difficulty, they offered me a small room in a run-down building for six hundred dollars a month. When I finally relocated there, I was exhausted. For about a month, I would wake up to do morning yoga, have breakfast, then go back to my room and sleep for most of the day. Part of me thought I was dying from some disease because I just couldn't move. I really had no idea how completely drained and exhausted I was after living in New York City for several years. Weeks passed before I woke up out of the grogginess and felt energized again. Eventually, I reached a point where I finally felt restored and better than ever. This experience confirmed something I often say: the body will heal itself by itself if given half a chance.

The moral of the story is that sometimes we know our battery is being drained and sometimes we don't, because on the bullet train of life, it's go, go, go 24/7. We are all distracted and chasing stuff in a highly stimulating world that becomes crazier every year. We give our energy away to other people so automatically that we don't even realize it. At the same time, our energy is also being drained by our environment.

♡ *What kinds of environments do you thrive in? What kinds of environments do you feel drained by?*

SEX AND PHYSICAL TOUCH

Sex is extremely beneficial to our health; it lowers blood pressure, boosts immunity, improves heart health, decreases anxiety and depression, relieves pain, enhances sleep, and reduces stress.[14] Sex can also be a spiritual experience: connecting with another person intimately on a profound emotional level and getting in touch with your body.

However, many people struggle with sex and intimacy. Sadly, I have spoken with a number of healers over the years who are survivors of sexual trauma. Traumatic sexual experiences often take a long time to recover from. For people who have been sexually violated, sex may become a source of stress rather than a stress reliever.

Some experience shame around sex because they were not properly educated about it from a young age. Many of us get our sex education from peers, movies, media, or porn. Others who grow up religious might be taught a very biased view of sex. Either way, plenty of us are not taught how to have a healthy relationship with our bodies and sexual desires. Because sex is so emphasized in our culture, if a person has physical, emotional, or mental barriers complicating their relationship with sex, it can significantly affect their self-esteem, confidence, and well-being.

The good news is there are many ways to experience nourishing physical touch beyond sex. For romantic partners, cuddling, hugging, kissing, and holding hands can provide calming, stress-relieving intimacy. For others, platonic physical intimacy—like receiving a healing massage, embracing a friend or child, or snuggling up with an animal companion—can calm the nervous system and improve mood and well-being.

With or without sex, physical intimacy through consensual touch is a fundamental human need. When honored respectfully, it eases tension in our bodies and nourishes our health. By expanding our understanding of intimacy beyond sex, we experience the benefits of caring physical connection in numerous positive ways.

♥ *How is your relationship with sex and physical touch?*

CHAPTER 11

MAP YOUR WAY TO WELL-BEING

♡

VISUALIZING THE LIFE YOU WANT IS empowering, because it puts you in the driver's seat. When your destination is clearly visible, you can map out how to get there. In this chapter, I'll go through some exercises and tools to help you design your future. Through intentional goal setting and visualizing your desired life, you'll start creating the reality you desire. Don't leave life up to chance—take ownership of your path. By giving yourself permission to daydream and make plans, you're planting seeds for real change. Now is the time to actively shape your trajectory instead of waiting for circumstances to improve.

TAKE THE LONG VIEW

When I used to coach people, I always ended sessions by giving my clients one or two recommendations. I developed this practice after seeing my teachers give clients ten or twenty recommendations at the end of sessions, only for the clients to come back and say they hadn't done any of them. So, I learned pretty quickly that people can only handle one or two manageable steps at a time. The thing is that bad habits take a long time to develop. So does burnout—it's the buildup of unaddressed stress over time. It makes sense that it would take a while to reverse some of those habits and start to replace them with new ones. Change takes time, but consistency creates progress.

When it comes to healing and improving your well-being, I encourage you to go slowly and take the long view. Think about change as an ongoing journey, not a destination. And try to be patient with yourself, even if you don't see dramatic results right away. It's kind of like investing in the stock market. If you check your portfolio every single day, some days you'll be up and others you'll be down, so you'll probably drive yourself a little mad. But if you invest consistently in quality funds and keep trusting the process, returns will build over time.

TIME TRAVEL EXERCISE

Albert Einstein once said that the past, present, and future are only illusions.[1] You're going to do an exercise now that enables you to travel through time, into the past and into the future. The purpose of this exercise is to get you thinking about your future in a serious way, so you can begin taking an active role in shaping your destiny rather than allowing life to happen to you.

Let's start by taking a trip down memory lane. Think back to your age and what your life was like ten years ago. Recall any issues or challenges you were dealing with at the time, whether in your relationships, career, health, or other aspects of your life. What emotions characterized that period?

Now, let's go back a bit further to when you were in elementary school. Recall the name of the school you went to and the names of a few people you were friends with. Then think about one or two of the teachers you had and what the experience of school was like for you. What was your inner state of being like at that point in your life compared to what it's like today? Think about your favorite childhood breakfast cereal or what you ate for lunch back then. Recall the name of the street you lived on.

Do you see how effectively you can travel through time and remember details within seconds, almost as if you were there? We have this ability to effectively travel through the past, like a supercomputer pulling up stored data. And if time is an illusion like Einstein said, we should be able to travel into the future as well.

In the second part of this exercise, you're going to look into your future. You get to go envision and shape it to your liking, just as if you were lucid dreaming. Sound good?

Before you can start mapping your way to well-being, you'll need to figure out your estimated life expectancy to help determine how many years you have left on this planet. Today, average life expectancy varies depending on gender, lifestyle factors, and where you live. In the US, the average life expectancy is around seventy-three for men and seventy-nine for women.[2] But leading a healthy lifestyle can significantly increase longevity. If you do not smoke, are not obese, and consume alcohol moderately, you can expect to live seven years longer than the general population.[3] And by the time you get to that age, average life expectancy will probably be even higher because of new innovations in healthcare and medicine.

So, go ahead and come up with a number to represent your estimated life expectancy. Then take your current age and subtract it from your life expectancy to determine how many years you have left. For example, if you are forty years old and your estimated life expectancy is one hundred, then you have sixty years left.

Do you have a clear plan for these years? Most people don't, and that's the problem. Lots of us think, "Well, who knows what's going to happen. I'll figure it out when I get there." But if you actually grasp that you're going to live for another two, three, or five decades, you might want to think about your life more strategically.

Life is a hundred-year marathon, not a hundred-meter dash. But as humans, we aren't very well equipped to think long term. This is one of the reasons our planet is struggling with climate change, among other issues. Most of us have trouble looking forward even five years from now, let alone fifty years from now. We go about our days focusing on the daily tasks and challenges life throws our way—the things we can check off our to-do lists. But when we focus only on short-term plans and fail to pace ourselves, we burn out. We lose sight of what matters most. We settle for less than what we really want.

So, here comes the fun part, where you get to figure out your long-term desires. I'm going to take you through some questions to help you envision your future. Write down your answers in a separate notebook or save them in a new document on your computer, because you will want to refer back to them for many years to come. This will become your road map for living a fuller, more intentional life.

1. What do you want to get done by the end of the day tomorrow? Create a list of any important priorities you have.

2. What do you want to get done by next weekend?

3. What do you want to get done by the end of next month?

4. What do you want to get done by the end of this year?

5. Now, write down the age you will be five years from now. Then write down the age of the most important people in your life—friends, partner, children, parents. Take their current ages and add five.

6. Now, answer the following questions:

   - Who do you want to be five years from now?

   - Where do you want to be living?

   - What do you want your career or income to look like?

   - What do you want your primary relationship to be like?

   - What do you want your other relationships to be like?

   - What do you want the central elements of your life to be by that time?

7. Repeat this visualization for ten and twenty years from now, if you wish.

I hope you are beginning to see how important it is to develop a vision for your life. Not having a map for your life is like trying to drive from Miami to Chicago without any sense of direction. You'll never get there. Maybe you'll end up in Kalamazoo instead. When you get to Kalamazoo, you might think, "Oh, this is great. I wasn't expecting to be in Kalamazoo, but isn't this interesting?" But at the end of your life, you might look back with regret.

Life is long. But it can go by quickly when you are not paying attention. Before you know it, you will be a decade older. And if you don't create a plan for yourself, the world will create one for you. Don't just drift wherever life takes you. Be intentional about the way you want to spend your energy and share your gifts with others. Life will still throw you surprises, but at least you'll have a clearer sense of direction.

If your plan is foggy right now, that's okay. You can fill in more specifics later. For now, just try to understand the importance of taking control of the direction you're going. Really consider what is important to you and what you want to manifest in your one precious life.

AMPLIFY YOUR RESOURCES

In the previous chapter, I asked you to assess how you are doing in different areas of life to help you reduce burnout and stress. You are now going to consider those same areas, but instead of assessing how you are *currently* doing in each one, you are going to describe your *ideal*. For example, maybe you wrote that you currently only take breaks when a client cancels at the last minute. Now, when you envision how you would *ideally* approach rest, you might write down the following:

Rest

- Schedule thirty minutes between each client session so I can recharge throughout my day.

- Lean into a sense of ease rather than anxiety when nothing is happening or planned.

- Learn the practice of parasympathetic reset: when I feel stressed, I will lie on the floor and look up at the ceiling, slow down my breathing, and do absolutely nothing.

Remember, this is about giving more to yourself, nourishing yourself, and making your life and work sustainable. Bring all the enthusiasm you want to envisioning your ideal in these areas—and try to keep it manageable and realistic. The point is *not* to stress yourself out trying to fit in all the things you need to do to de-stress yourself! Some of your answers may not be tasks to fit in but attitudes you'd like to cultivate, ways you'd like to feel, or more enjoyable methods for the things you're already doing.

What does your ideal look like in the following areas?

- Bodywork
- Physical activity

- Mindfulness
- Purpose and meaning
- Joy and play
- Rest
- Sleep
- Financial self-care
- Mutually supportive relationships
- Environment
- Sex and physical touch

Reflection

Using the lists of ideals you just created, decide what is most important to you at this time. What areas do you want to prioritize and improve first? What are the initial steps you need to take?

What people, groups, and resources do you need to support you? List some individuals, groups, or resources you can turn to for support in creating your ideal life.

SMART GOALS

As the proverb goes, "A goal without a plan is just a wish." Setting SMART goals—specific, measurable, achievable, relevant, and time-bound—can help you turn big dreams into reality. Start by identifying your larger goals (e.g., swapping urban life for small town living, or starting your own business), then break these down into smaller, actionable steps, and add deadlines to make them more concrete and manageable. For example, "start a yoga studio" becomes "research locations," "draft a business plan," "find funding," etc.

Regularly revisit and adjust your SMART goals as you move toward your bigger vision, and stay motivated and accountable by tracking progress along the way. SMART goals transform vague dreams into clear roadmaps. With focus and discipline, you can make stuff happen that once seemed out of reach.

Ready to create SMART goals of your own?

1. List your top three goals for the next year.

2. Break these goals down into smaller, actionable SMART goals.

3. Reflect. Are the things that seemed out of reach starting to look more attainable? Are you feeling more empowered to take action?

CHAPTER 12
FITTING OUT

♡

A S HEALERS, LOTS OF US ALREADY FEEL uncomfortably different from other people, so we avoid standing out and put our energy into fitting in. Some healers dress conservatively, get nine-to-five jobs, and participate in conventions that don't align with what's in their hearts. There is so much emphasis in our culture on belonging that many would rather hide who they truly are than dare to be different. But resisting being true to ourselves affects our ability to heal and help others.

Fitting out is exactly what it sounds like—the opposite of fitting in.[1] It means having the courage to be who we are, even if it makes us stand out or draws judgment. Fitting out is an act of healing. When we stop conforming and start expressing our true essence, we feel more empowered and alive. The freedom we gain from fitting out allows us to help others fit out, too.

> ## HEALER HIGHLIGHT
>
> **"I'm in the last two weeks of my corporate job as an IT manager before I make a huge shift and become the new owner of a yoga studio. It feels like a brave step to trust that I'll be okay when I'm doing the work that's in alignment with my inner knowing and true purpose. For so long, I've toed the line and done what was expected of me, trying to fit in where I never really belonged. Very soon, I will have a new work home where my livelihood can become connected to my heart. I am excited and nervous all at once!"—SARAH from Florida**

We all have a deep inner knowing, though many of us are afraid to trust it. Instead, we rely on external influencers and so-called experts to tell us how to live. It takes constant effort to untrain our minds—to learn to be guided by our own intuition rather than other people's expectations. But we gain back our zest for life when we start living on our own terms, trusting our bodies and ourselves. Being bold and brave—coming out and being who you authentically are—can be a real gift to others, especially in a time when not many people are prepared to do that.

I encourage you to experiment with fitting out. Challenge social pressures to conform by acting more in alignment with your authentic self. Surround yourself with people who embrace your individuality as you take the risks necessary to move your life forward. Through exploring new ways of being, you'll gain confidence and strength. Then, at the end of your amazing journey, you can look back and say, "I really lived my best life possible."

THE AGILITY MINDSET

I have noticed a common thread amongst healers: we tend to stay in careers or relationships that leave us unfulfilled or communities we've outgrown. As someone who has reinvented myself many times, I understand the challenges of changing course when your current path no longer nourishes you. Change usually feels uncomfortable and scary. But resisting change can trap us in burnout. When we embrace change and uncertainty, we give ourselves permission to discover where our spirit wants to soar next. With an agility mindset and willingness to try new things, we can skillfully lean into transitions. By listening to our inner wisdom and honoring our core values, we're free to walk an authentic path that nourishes us, so that we may continue to nourish others.

People have told me that I have a remarkable capacity for being agile. This is how I was able to pick up and move from Canada to New York to start a school. It's been a theme throughout my life: I am not afraid to try things or to shift directions. For example, I tried starting an organic restaurant once. Then, when I realized it wasn't for me, I said, "Okay, I'm done with this," and moved on to something else.

An agility mindset means staying alert to what matters in the present and adjusting as you take in new information. It's waking up in the morning and saying, "This is Day One. Nothing in the past matters. Who am I going to be today? What am I going to invent?"

When I first started IIN, I didn't have a business plan. Creating the school was just a thing I wanted to do to meet more like-minded people. I wanted to create a community. And I was learning that most people's health concerns come down to the food they eat—and the energy and passion they feel in their lives on a soul level. I figured if I could educate people to educate their friends, family, and clients, the world would become a better place. I could start a ripple effect to bring more consciousness into the world.

In its first year, the school faced a lot of financial challenges. The government didn't want the school to exist. I would go to court hearings with registered dieticians and the American Psychological Association. They were concerned that I was putting people into the healthcare system after just twelve months of studying. There was no language to describe what I was teaching and doing, so I had to make things up as I went. Originally, the school trained students to become *health counselors*, but the Association said we couldn't use the term "counselors." So, I said, "How about health coaching? Is that okay?" And they said that was fine.

I developed a lot of unique wording to be able to keep moving the ball forward. It was kind of a miracle that the government and these big organizations eventually saw the light. They empowered the school. Now, the Institute for Integrative Nutrition is licensed by New York State. And health coaching, which I am credited with inventing, is a $13 billion global industry. None of this would exist if I wasn't willing to be agile, come up with creative solutions, and overcome obstacles as they arose.

To be agile, we must be comfortable with fitting out. We must be willing to invent behavior, even if that behavior takes us outside the box of what other people expect from us. When you are agile, you don't reach a roadblock and quit. You pivot and find a way to keep going.

♥ *Can you think of any creative solutions for a problem you are currently dealing with?*

BE BAD

After many years of seeing clients and talking to students, I noticed that "being good" is a high priority for people. A lot of people have strict rules they live by—rules for eating, exercising, and countless other things. They want to be good for their bosses, clients, spouses, partners, social media, and others, so they hold themselves to standards of goodness they think they need to meet to gain acceptance and approval.

I distinctly remember one student who was trying to lose weight. She knew avocados were healthy, but had a phobia around eating fat, so she would cut an avocado into seven pieces and have only one piece per day. I finally said to her, "Why don't you be bad and just eat an entire avocado at once?" At first, she looked at me like I had just suggested something illegal. But she came back the next day beaming and said, "I ate the whole avocado, and I feel great!" Today, she is inspiring many people as a healer and health coach.

Another student told me she was waking up at 5:30 each morning to meditate, even though that meant getting only six hours of sleep each night. I asked why she didn't just sleep an extra thirty minutes instead of meditating, and this ended up being a better decision for her health. People get so caught up in what they are *supposed to be doing* that they neglect their own basic needs.

I started doing an exercise with students to help them realize that life isn't just about pleasing other people; it's also about pleasing and taking care of yourself. The assignment I gave was to go home and do one *bad* thing. Then, the next day, we would compare notes, and the person who did the "baddest" thing would win a prize. To be clear, I wasn't encouraging anyone to rob a bank, cheat on their spouse, or do anything dangerous or illegal. Being bad, as I explained it, could mean deleting all of your unread emails, skipping the gym, or ordering the most expensive item on the menu at a restaurant—anything that goes against people's habitual rule-following. The purpose of the exercise was to put people in charge of their lives. Sometimes, we think we need to be perfect to be in control. But it is inauthentic to live life pretending to be perfect. People are not perfect. And when we become too obedient, life can get pretty dull. Sometimes, taking risks is necessary in order to experience joy and move our lives forward.

I'll never forget the time I did the Be Bad exercise with students in Miami Beach, and these guys jumped into a fountain near the shops on Lincoln Road and started dancing in the fountain. Another group of students decided to break into the liquor cabinet at the venue where classes were being held. When I came back from lunch, they had a whole bar open and were handing out free drinks. The venue wanted to kick us out after that, so I had to beg them to let us stay. We had four more weekends left, so I had to leave a big deposit and pay extra for insurance.

These students took the concept a little too far, but the point is that many of us need permission to deviate from the safe, contained realities we are living in. Having that permission can be really freeing. It allows people to tap into their spontaneous desires and test themselves in new ways.

I have tears in my eyes just writing about this, because it is deeply moving to witness what people are capable of when they wake up to the present moment rather than unconsciously going through the motions of life. The next time you're stuck in a rut, try doing one bad thing a day. Sometimes, we need to be reminded of what it's like to have fun.

♡ *What's one bad thing you can give yourself permission to do in the next twenty-four hours? How can you add more bad behavior into your life?*

BIO-INDIVIDUALITY

Bio-individuality is one of the key ideas I developed at the beginning of IIN. There is no one-size-fits-all approach to a healthy lifestyle. Every person has unique needs and preferences, which evolve over time. The more we try new things, the more new information we learn about ourselves. Throughout our lives, we should be consistently assessing ourselves and what we need to feel healthier and happier.

The concept of bio-individuality came about when I was in the process of reading countless books about diet, food, and nutrition. I realized that many theories and ideas about healthy eating conflicted with one another. One expert suggested that humans should be eating meat and dairy, while another said that humans should never eat meat or dairy and we should all be vegan.

This got me thinking. Eventually, through meditation, I arrived at the idea that one person's food is another person's poison. There is no single right way of eating—or of doing anything else, for that matter. Every body is biochemically different, and what works for you today may not even work for you tomorrow. You could find a diet that makes you feel great for a while, but that same diet could make you feel sick five years from now. The same goes for other areas of life: you might thrive in a certain environment, relationship, or career in one season of life, but in time, that may change.

I'm including bio-individuality within this chapter on fitting out to remind you that humans are not designed to all be the same. Although the things that set us apart from other people often bring us shame, it is completely normal for there to be variation among members of the same species. The more we embrace these differences in ourselves, the more we can empower others to do the same.

♡ *If you paid more attention to your unique bio-individual makeup than any general theory or prescription for well-being, are there any habits or practices you would change?*

TRUST MORE, DO LESS

As the director of a school, at some point I learned to hire the right people and trust them to do their jobs rather than trying to do everything myself. Some of us get into roles where we are expected to be the primary decision-makers of a company or a family. But realistically, there is only so much one person can manage. We get decision fatigue when we try to handle too much, and we can grow resentful of the people around us if we are not being supported.

To this day, when someone asks me a question and I have no idea what the answer is, I'll say, "Just do what you think is best." This is my way of empowering the people around me to be more self-sufficient and trust in their capability to make decisions. It is not always easy to maintain this attitude, as it requires surrendering to the possibility that things will not get done exactly the way I would do them. But by giving up a little bit of control and trusting the right people, I accomplish a lot more than I could alone.

Empowering people to have more self-efficacy was one of my intentions when I started the IIN. I wanted to inspire students to trust in the wisdom of their bodies and to take their health into their own hands rather than relying entirely on the healthcare system. I trained students to become health coaches who could inspire self-efficacy in their clients as well.

Many people today are looking for a quick fix—someone

to tell them exactly what to eat, how to exercise, and what to do to be healthy. But most would benefit more from self-connection and experimenting with what works for them as individuals. IIN's Health Coach Training Program teaches health coaches to let the client lead, trusting them as the expert on their own life instead of telling them what to do. The health coach is the "guide on the side" rather than the "sage on the stage," which empowers clients to take responsibility for their own health and happiness.

Do you get where I'm going with this? It's not a healer's job to change, control, or force anyone to see something they aren't willing to see. When we overfunction in relationships—with clients, employees, family members, partners, or anyone else in our lives—we may think we deserve a gold medal for running the show and doing everything to the highest standard. But what we are actually doing is exhausting ourselves while disempowering others from rising to their potential.

I had a client many years ago with the tendency to overfunction. As a busy career mom with a thriving wellness clinic, she felt overwhelmed trying to juggle work, kids, and everything else, and she felt her husband wasn't helping enough. She was agitated, anxious, and resentful, and often ended up verbally attacking him. So, I gave her some homework.

"Why don't you try doing less?" I suggested. At first, she had a hard time understanding what I meant.

"Like, not do the laundry and the dishes and clean up after the kids?" she said.

I nodded.

"But if I don't do it, no one will," she said.

"And?" I replied.

"And then everything will fall apart."

"Will everything actually fall apart?" I asked. "Or will there just be dishes in the sink, clothes unwashed, and some extra mess around the house? What if, instead of doing these chores with resentment, you go rest and put your feet up instead?"

Finally, she paused to consider this. She was resistant but finally agreed.

"Okay, I'll try it," she said. "But only for a week."

A week later my client returned, and I could see a dramatic shift in her. She was more relaxed. When I asked her how her week went, she told me about the miraculous thing that happened. When she allowed herself to rest, her husband stepped up. He emptied the dishwasher each day when he got home from work. Over the weekend he did two loads of laundry, and he took the kids out for the entire day on Sunday.

"That sounds like progress," I said. "Do you see how by pulling back, you made space for your husband to support you more?"

"Yeah," she said, "and it probably helped that I made an effort to be kinder to him."

In time, my client and her husband were able to work together to create more balance in their relationship. And my client's commitment to trusting more and doing less was a big step in the couple's healing.

Often, anxious healers and caregivers overfunction because they don't trust other people to support them. They do everything themselves to feel in control, but then they resent the people around them who seem freer. It feels counterintuitive, but sometimes getting what we want means letting go and seeing what happens.

Letting go of control can be hard if you're not used to it. It requires vulnerability to allow someone else to drive the car while you take a nap in the passenger seat, meta-phorically speaking. But allowing yourself to be cared for will deepen your relationships, relieve stress, and let you experience more freedom. If receiving help is difficult, remember how good it feels to be useful and needed; sometimes others want to feel that way, too! Reframe receiving as a form of giving if that makes it easier to accept support.

♡ *How do you overfunction in relationships? How do your overfunctioning behaviors help you avoid vulner-ability? What is one area where you could benefit from trusting more and doing less?*

SHIFTING FROM CONSUMER TO LEADER

If you've ever been tempted to try the latest fad diet because everyone else was doing it, then you know what it's like to be influenced by what is popular at any given moment. This is herd mentality, and to some extent, it's human instinct to follow the crowd rather than thinking independently. But when we act this way, we become passive consumers rather than active creators. To make a difference, we need to shift from being consumers to leaders—to resist conformity, question the status quo, and create our own reality based on inner truth.

I always found it fascinating that many students enrolled in IIN's Health Coach Training Program because they themselves had a health issue that couldn't be resolved by a doctor. They took their health into their own hands and, by changing their diet or lifestyle, healed their issue themselves. And that experience was like a crack in the cosmic egg for them: the moment they woke up and realized they couldn't trust the healthcare system like they'd thought they could. From there, they would start questioning other things, trusting less in external sources and more in the wisdom of their bodies.

As a healer, you are likely more self-aware than most. Instead of gathering more data and information, you will probably benefit more from trusting what you already know. I guarantee you that even on your worst days, you have gifts and resources that others don't. Find communities that will listen to you, and let your divine wisdom guide you.

Remember, you don't have to be perfect to change the world. Just show up fully and authentically. If you tend toward perfectionism, see if you can challenge yourself to be *good enough*. This is what it means to be in charge of your own life. You get to make the rules and decide what being a leader means to you. You get to decide whose opinions to listen to and whose opinions to ignore.

Over time, healers may make a more conscious, compassionate world by leading through example. Start exploring moving away from herd mentality and stand out. It can be challenging at first but will ultimately feel more and more empowering. When we stand in our power, we attract others doing the same, which makes us stronger together.

CHAPTER 13

THE POWER OF COMMUNITY

♡

T HERE IS A LOT OF CONFUSION IN THE
world right now. Many of the institutions that used to
make up the fabric of society are dissipating or fragment-
ing. Fewer people are religious than in the past. Fewer
people are getting married, and there is less emphasis on
the family unit. So, what values do we live by now? What
is governing us?

The fact that things are changing is a good thing. People
have more freedom today to explore themselves independent of systems, traditions, and codes of behavior. More
people have the freedom to choose who they are and what
they stand for.

But with the disintegration of traditional values, there
are also things we have lost. I remember eating dinner

with my family at six o'clock every night when I was a kid. This meal was the center point of the day, when I knew I was going to sit down at a table with my mom, dad, and brother. We were a unified, cohesive family. It was a time to rest, reset, and connect with one another. Today, families rarely sit down at the dinner table together. They're too busy. Instead, the home has become more like a hotel, where family members come and go as they please. And with less emphasis on religion, fewer people are engaging in spiritual practices that connect them to a larger community.

In addition to being more segregated from one another, we are also more divided than ever. There is tremendous pressure to choose a side when it comes to social and political issues. People are quick to criticize one another's opinions and bully each other from behind screens. As a result, our mental, emotional, and physical health is suffering. Many people lack a sense of purpose and belonging. Our souls are yearning for deeper meaning and connection. It's like we're on the brink of a spiritual crisis.

Where do we go from here? As our values as a society continue to evolve, where are we headed? What should we strive for? The answer that's obvious to me is that we need to find new ways to come together. We need to redevelop our sense of community. Without tribes and communities, we would not have survived this long as a species. So, what's next? What things do we need to rediscover, and what do we need to rebuild?

WHY COMMUNITY IS CRUCIAL

Our individualist society teaches us that we should be dependent as infants and children and then mature into autonomous adults. But even as adults, we have a natural, primal need to be connected to other people. It is not something we grow out of, and it doesn't make us needy. As Esther Perel said, "The quality of your life ultimately depends on the quality of your relationships."[1] We can only get so far on our own. When we have the support of a loving community, we are stronger. We are in a better position to heal ourselves and society.

There is a reason animals and birds migrate far distances in large groups rather than going it alone. It is natural to take refuge in others for a sense of belonging and, in some cases, protection. Animals are more secure when they move together. The same is true for human beings. When we move toward a shared goal with others who are walking the same path, we exchange energy with those people in a way that nourishes us and restores our balance. In this mutual exchange, transformation and healing become possible. Every individual who is part of the group benefits from the group's collective strength, consciousness, and insight.

This is why community is so crucial. Humans are not meant to accomplish big tasks alone. We are meant to work together. When we attempt to solve issues on our own, we inevitably encounter mental resistance. We get tired and overwhelmed by the limitations of our minds. But when we share our burdens and our gifts with a supportive community, we feel less lonely. We find ways to conquer things together and gain the confidence to slow down, so that we can be mindful about the choices we make.

It's especially important for healers to build community with each other given the unique stressors and emotional loads they carry, and because many healers work independently and remotely, without much daily support. Partners, kids, parents, and friends might not get what you are going through, but colleagues in helping professions are more likely to understand. In a supportive community, healers can give and receive compassion, process trauma, and restore depleted reserves. They can also share insights on healthy boundaries, balance, and avoiding burnout. Together, healers can uplift each other as they work to uplift humanity.

However powerful you are as an individual, when you stand alongside a supportive community of other individuals all working toward a similar goal, you will raise your game. You will gain access to that community's collective wisdom and resources. You will open your mind to fresh ideas and perspectives. And you will find that your strengths and weaknesses are balanced by the group, so that you feel more stable as an individual.

♡ *What groups or communities are you already a part of? Are they rooted in values or causes you believe in? What groups or communities would you like to be a part of that you are not currently involved with? What is one community-based activity (e.g., a weekly meditation workshop, a Meetup group, volunteer work) you could see yourself participating in on a regular basis?*

HEALING WITH OTHER HEALERS

So much of my life's work has been about bringing like-minded people together—healers and others who share a conscious vision for the future. This is because I believe in my heart of hearts that together we are stronger. If I can help five people heal, and if those five people each help five more people heal, that's thirty people. That ripple effect soon reaches a hundred people, then a thousand, and so on.

So many people on this planet just need someone to listen to them and help them process their emotions, and healers are no exception. In fact, healers need this sort of support the most—yet it's hard to come by. Most people want to give us advice or information rather than sit with us in our pain. There are some people who have never felt what it's like to have someone listen to them with full attention.

This is why health coaching is mostly about allowing the client to speak freely, so they can get whatever they need to say off their chest. As the client shares what is in their heart, they start listening to themselves, and they usually get better without a huge amount of input from the coach. The coach just has to know how to ask the right questions—ones that prompt the client to open up about areas that are painful for them.

When I started health coaching, I was astonished at how supported people felt just by having me listen to them. I was basically being paid to sit and meditate. Breathe in, breathe out. Ask high-mileage questions. Don't give too much advice, because people mostly just need someone to witness and hold space for them while they process whatever they need to process. It's kind of like when a toddler falls down and starts crying while learning to walk—you don't have to do much because you know that a few minutes later, they are going to be just fine. As adults, we aren't so different. We are those same toddlers, just a few years older. We still need a safe space to unwind and process what we've been through. We need to allow our emotions to run their course because that is how stress moves out of our system.

As healers, this is something we can do for one another. We can practice active listening and holding space for other healers and then gain the therapeutic benefits that come with it. You can do this by partnering up with other healers in your community, starting weekly or monthly healing circles, or joining healing-centered groups that already exist. There is something really beneficial about connecting with like-minded people in a group setting and being accountable to those people. It can be even more therapeutic than individual therapy.

The more you practice active listening, the more you will see other people as reflections of yourself. While they are learning from you, you are learning from them. As we relate to one another, we become bonded in ways that break down barriers. This is the greatest gift—getting to realize that we are all connected through our shared human experience. We might wear different clothing and come from different backgrounds, but what we have in common is so much greater than our differences.

As a healer, it is especially important for you to connect with other healers who understand your specific struggles and can relate to what you're going through. These are the people you want by your side as you go through life's trials and tribulations. Unlike those in your life who feel entitled to your time, energy, and resources, fellow healers are people you can build mutually supportive relationships with. Together, we can hold one another accountable and validate one another's experiences.

SURROUND YOURSELF WITH MENTORS

You have probably heard the saying, "Show me your friends, and I'll show you your future." The people we spend the most time with have a significant impact on our lives. If your friends eat junk food and complain a lot, you'll probably eat junk food and complain a lot. If your friends like to hike and do outdoor activities, you'll probably hike and do outdoor activities. We are all born limitless, then we develop limiting beliefs as we grow older. If you want to grow as a person, the goal is not to surround yourself with people who reinforce your familiar, limiting beliefs but with friends and mentors who inspire you to grow. These should be people who share your mission and values— people you can learn from.

Throughout my life, I have surrounded myself with mentors I wanted to learn from. Over a period of several years, I spent a good amount of time with Michio Kushi, the creator of modern macrobiotics, who launched the organic natural food movement. He created some of the first natural food stores and taught that food was the key to health, happiness, and world peace. I sat in on his counseling sessions and traveled with him to Japan. I learned a lot from him: what to do and what not to do. I am forever grateful to him for his wisdom and passion.

I encourage you to find ways to connect with thought leaders and people who inspire you. Try to spend time with these people in person if you can. Or follow them on social media. Read their books and watch their videos. When you expose yourself to people who interest you, who you admire, you will gain a clearer understanding of your own health and happiness.

If you prefer to have a mentor you can work with more closely, I suggest starting with your local community and existing social network. Seek out people who have had success in an area you are interested in learning more about, then reach out to them and ask if they would be willing to mentor you. You may offer to pay potential mentors or take them out to lunch in exchange for sharing their expertise. You could also volunteer for a thought leader or business in exchange for industry experience and mentorship. Mentors who work with you closely empower you to identify your strengths and gain clarity around your goals. They will also provide accountability and connect you with other helpful people and opportunities.

If you need help finding potential mentors, you could attend conferences, networking events, trade shows, and industry meetups to connect with people in specific industries. Or you could search for groups or individuals online that offer personalized mentoring. Meetup.com allows you to search for groups and events based on keywords and location. Some groups meet online and others meet in person. LinkedIn is a great resource for finding mentors as it allows you to search for people using keywords. On LinkedIn, you can see people's work experience, job titles, and industries they are involved in. You may also join a mentorship platform like MentorCruise, GrowthMentor, or Clarity. These platforms charge fees, but the investment could be worth it if you gain knowledge and resources that help you progress forward in your personal life or career.

Personally, I like having a group of mentors I can turn to when I need help thinking through an issue or making an important decision. Some people would call this a mastermind group. You can easily create your own mastermind group in your community or online by gathering a few peers who have expertise in an area you are interested in. These should be people who know more than you do about a certain topic or at least have a similar amount of knowledge and skills they can share with you. You can then decide to meet as a group however frequently you want, either virtually or in person. Or if you prefer to have support at your fingertips, you can start a group chat using any number of messaging platforms and create a forum for group members to ask questions whenever they need input or advice.

♡ *Do you surround yourself with people you can learn from and grow with—people you consider mentors? Name three thought leaders you look up to (e.g., authors, bloggers, industry influencers you follow on social media). What is it about each of these individuals that interests you? What key players would you include in your ideal mastermind group?*

COLLECTIVE CONNECTION

Have you ever felt a buzz after seeing your favorite band in concert? After going to a big sports game? How about after a group fitness class? If you know what I'm talking about, then you have experienced the collective catharsis that happens when we share energy and emotions with a crowd of people who have come together for the same cause. It is for this reason that many religious and spiritual rituals involve singing, chanting, breathing, meditation, or synchronized movement with a group. When we participate in these practices, we coregulate with strangers in a way that calms our nervous systems. We feel connected to something sacred and meaningful, and we are reminded of our shared humanity.

It can be particularly healing to connect with groups of strangers over shared feelings of grief and pain. Research has proven that social support enhances resilience to stress and decreases the impact of PTSD.[2] Sometimes just being in the presence of others who can relate to your experiences, even if you don't talk about those experiences, is comforting. Their shared knowing can help normalize what you are going through. For example, after the Holocaust, it was therapeutic for many survivors to spend time with other survivors, even if all they did was play cards together or share meals. The same goes for soldiers who return from combat with PTSD; it is healthy to maintain relationships with other veterans, since most people in society can't relate to their experiences, which can feel isolating.

Collective connection can be an especially great way to be with others if you are highly introverted. There are plenty of creative ways to heal and bond with other people over shared interests and experiences that don't involve lots of talking.

♥ *Do you intentionally seek out opportunities for collective connection? If not, what are some ways you can increase the amount of collective connection in your life?*

THE HEAL THE HEALER LIVE EXPERIENCE

As a way to help you connect with other healers, I am developing a live component to this book: the Heal the Healer Live Experience. It is important to me, in addition to writing about all of this, to help facilitate in-person healing opportunities using the platform I have created.

The Heal the Healer Live Experience will be an opportunity for you to connect with myself and other healers at various locations in the United States and abroad. The mission of Heal the Healer Live aligns with the mission of this book: to support wellness workers and caregivers who feel emotionally exhausted, overworked, and overwhelmed, and to inspire collective healing. I hope you will join me in person to expand the Heal the Healer movement. You can visit my website, joshuarosenthal.me, for details and updates.

Together, we are stronger.

CONCLUSION

♡

$\mathbf{A}$ S YOU LOOK TO THE FUTURE, IMAGINE WHAT could be possible on a global level if healers were healthy, happy, and empowered. When we support one another to rest and heal, so that our hearts and minds can operate at full capacity, our potential is truly limitless. Do you see how much greater our impact would be if we tapped into our collective wisdom and resources? Whether we like it or not, we are all interconnected. This is why we cannot fully heal ourselves by ourselves; we must also rely on one another.

Allowing others to support us and carry some of our responsibilities and emotions is not easy. Healers are highly conscientious and tend to give to others without expecting much in return. But when we resist being cared for, we starve ourselves emotionally. We deny ourselves a big part of the human experience. It is okay to be vulnerable, to lean on others who are stable enough to give us strength.

This work of healing requires a lot of effort. I know many people get overwhelmed once they start analyzing the things they have been conditioned to believe from a young age. There is grief in waking up and realizing that a lot of what we have been taught has prevented us from living up to our full potential. But it is better to face the truth now than continue living in denial. Yes, awareness can make you regret the years you spent in a relationship, job, or other situation that didn't serve you. Once you know better, it becomes more difficult to look back on your past decisions. But this is why it's important to practice self-compassion and forgiveness, and to surrender along the way.

I also recognize that fitting out can be lonely. When you step out of the roles that others expect of you and do the work to heal, your former communities may no longer feel authentic to you. This is why I created the Heal the Healer community, to support you as you push against the current and move toward positive transformation.

Now is the time to give yourself permission to color outside the lines. Experiment with new ways of being. Tap into your resilience. Take a leap of faith. Walking this path isn't about being perfect; it's about being brave. So, listen to the voice of truth that lives inside you—even when it goes against social expectations. Trust yourself. Embrace your unique gifts. Make space for everything that is possible.

Most importantly, remember that healing takes time. You didn't become numb, overwhelmed, and exhausted overnight. You operate this way because of years of conditioning, so it's going to take some time before you start feeling better. There is no quick fix, only a slow unraveling and reweaving. Your only job is to stay committed to the process of rebuilding your relationship with yourself. Give yourself grace and time to rest. Recognize the progress you make, even it's only a small shift at first. Surround yourself with people that lift you up. And remember, the most important thing you can do to heal the world is to heal yourself.

RESOURCES

For details about the heal the healer live experience, sign up for my mailing list at joshuarosenthal.me.

GENERAL

Aging Care Caregiver Forum
agingcare.com/caregiver-forum

ARCH National Respite Network and Resource Center
archrespite.org

ART International—Authentic Relating Training
authenticrelating.co

Authentic Revolution
authrev.org

The Center for Nonviolent Communication
cnvc.org

Compassion Fatigue Awareness Project
compassionfatigue.org

Family Caregiver Alliance

caregiver.org

The Highly Sensitive Person

hsperson.com

NVC Academy

nvcacademy.com

US Department of Health and Human Services—Resources for Caregivers

hhs.gov/programs/providers-and-facilities
/resources-for-caregivers/index.html

Vicarious Trauma Institute

vicarioustrauma.com

HOTLINES/HELPLINES

Crisis Text Line

crisistextline.org

* Text HOME to 741741. Text message-based hotline providing support to people experiencing a crisis. Available 24/7.

988 Suicide & Crisis Lifeline

988lifeline.org

* The 988 Lifeline provides 24/7, free and confidential support for people in distress, prevention and crisis

resources for you or your loved ones, and best practices for professionals in the United States. Available 24/7.

OUTSOURCING

Instacart
instacart.com

TaskRabbit
taskrabbit.com

Thumbtack
thumbtack.com

FINDING MENTORS

Meetup
meetup.com

LinkedIn
linkedin.com

MentorCruise
mentorcruise.com

Growth Mentor
growthmentor.com

Clarity
clarity.fm

BOOKS

Authentic Relating: A Guide to Rich, Meaningful, Nourishing Relationships by Ryel Kestano

Burnout: The Secret to Unlocking the Stress Cycle by Emily Nagoski, PhD, and Amelia Nagoski

The Conscious Caregiver by Linda Abbit

The Empath's Survival Guide: Life Strategies for Sensitive People by Judith Orloff

Set Boundaries, Find Peace: A Guide to Reclaiming Yourself by Nedra Glover Tawwab

Healing Secondary Trauma: Proven Strategies for Caregivers and Professionals to Manage Stress, Anxiety, and Compassion Fatigue by Trudy Gilbert-Eliot

Nonviolent Communication: A Language of Life by Marshall Rosenberg

NOTES

INTRODUCTION

1. Margarita Tartakovsky, "Healing Burnout and Compassion Fatigue as a Helping Professional," PsychCentral.com, January 8, 2022, psychcentral.com/blog/healing-burnout-compassion-fatigue-helping-professional#1.
2. World Health Organization, "COVID-19 Pandemic Triggers 25% Increase in Prevalence of Anxiety and Depression Worldwide," March 2, 2022, www.who.int/news/item/02-03-2022-covid-19-pandemic-triggers-25-increase-in-prevalence-of-anxiety-and-depression-worldwide.
3. Tamara Hayford and David Austin, "Prescription Drugs: Spending, Use, Prices," Congressional Budget Office, January 2022, www.cbo.gov/publication/57772; Andrew Gallant, "A Growing Number of Americans Report Taking Prescription Medications Daily," CivicScience, January 11, 2023, https://civicscience.com/a-growing-number-of-americans-report-taking-prescription-medications-daily/.
4. Brendan Martin, Nicole Kaminski-Ozturk, Charlie O'Hara, and Richard Smiley (NCSBN), "Examining the Impact of the COVID-19 Pandemic on Burnout and Stress Among U.S. Nurses," *Journal of Nursing Regulation*, April 13, 2023, www.ncsbn.org/public-files/examining_impact_of_covid_on_nurse_stress.pdf.

1: HEALER BURNOUT

1. "Cultivating Resilience from Stress, Burnout, and PTSD: Building Teams and Leaders." University of Virginia School of Medicine Center for Appreciative Practice. January 3, 2023. Retrieved from

https://cap.med.virginia.edu/articles/cultivating-resilience-from
-stress-burnout-and-ptsd-building-teams-and-leaders.

2. I. L. McCann and L. A. Pearlman, "Vicarious Traumatization: A
Framework for Understanding the Psychological Effects of Working with Victims," *Journal of Trauma Stress* 3 (1990): 131–149.

3. THE HEALER PERSONALITY

1. Jerome Kagan and Nancy Snidman, *The Long Shadow of
Temperament* (Cambridge, MA: Harvard University Press, 2004).

2. Elaine N. Aron, *The Highly Sensitive Person: How to Thrive When
the World Overwhelms You* (New York: Broadway Books, 1997).

3. Elaine Aron, "The Highly Sensitive Child," Highly Sensitive
Person, accessed May 10, 2023, https://hsperson.com/books
/the-highly-sensitive-child.

4. Myers and Briggs Foundation, "Sensing or Intuition," accessed
May 10, 2023, www.myersbriggs.org/my-mbti-personality-type
/mbti-basics/sensing-or-intuition.htm.

5. Molly Owens, "The Intuitive's Guide to Getting Along with
Sensors," Truity, September 28, 2015, www.truity.com/blog
/intuitives-guide-getting-along-sensors.

4. WHAT NEEDS TO BE HEALED

1. Wikipedia, "Wounded Healer," accessed October 5, 2023,
en.wikipedia.org/wiki/Wounded_healer.

2. Center for Addiction and Mental Health, "Trauma," accessed May
10, 2023, www.camh.ca/en/health-info
/mental-illness-and-addiction-index/trauma.

3. Nicole Harris, "What Is Parentification? Spotting the Warning
Signs," Parents, December 31, 2022, www.parents.com/kids
/development/what-is-parentification-spotting-the-warning
-signs-and-how-to-let-kids-be-kids.

4. Sharon Martin, "When Kids Have to Act Like Adults,"
PsychCentral.com, January 31, 2020, https://psychcentral.com
/blog/imperfect/2020/01/when-kids-have-to-act-like-adults.

5. Joy DeGruy, *Post Traumatic Slave Syndrome: America's Legacy of
Enduring Injury and Healing* (Joy DeGruy Publications Inc., 2017).

5. THE SOCIAL FORCES THAT SHAPE US

1. Neel Chowdhury, "In Singapore, Finding Peace among the Pain of Thaipusam," *Time*, February 9, 2023, http://content.time.com /time/world/article/0,8599,2106461,00.html.

2. Kendra Cherry, "What Is a Collectivist Culture," Verywell Mind, November 8, 2022, www.verywellmind.com /what-are-collectivistic-cultures-2794962.

3. "Integrative Nutrition's Secret to Total Health: Bio-Individuality," Institute for Integrative Nutrition, August 2016, www.integrativenutrition.com/blog/2016/08 /integrative-nutrition-s-secret-to-total-health-bio-individuality.

4. Bureau of Labor Statistics, US Department of Labor, Occupational Outlook Handbook, Home Health and Personal Care Aides, www.bls.gov/ooh/healthcare/home-health-aides-and-personal-care-aides.htm

7. HEAL YOUR CHILDHOOD WOUNDS

1. "What Is Rolfing and How Is It Different from Massage?" Cleveland Clinic, October 11, 2022, https://health.clevelandclinic.org /rolfing-massage-benefits.

2. Cassie Green, "How to Improve Resilience in Caregiving," Multicultural Caregiving, accessed October 11, 2023, https://multiculturalcaregiving.net how-to-improve-resilience -in-caregiving/.

3. Kristin Neff, "The Space Between Self-Esteem and Self-Compassion," TEDx Talk, February 6, 2013, www.youtube.com /watch?v=IvtZBUSplr4.

4. Green, "How to Improve Resilience in Caregiving."

5. R. Dotinga, "Half of Americans Over 50 Are Now Caregivers," *U.S. News & World Report*, November 3, 2022, www.usnews.com/news/health-news/articles/2022-11-03 /half-of-americans-over-50-are-now-caregivers.

6. Green, "How to Improve Resilience in Caregiving."

7. Erika Stoerkel, "What Is a Strength-Based Approach? (Incl. Examples and Tools)," PositivePsychology.com, March 12, 2019, https://positivepsychology.com/strengths-based-interventions/.

8. ASSERT YOUR BOUNDARIES

1. Brené Brown, *Dare to Lead: Brave Work, Tough Conversations, Whole Hearts* (New York: Random House, 2018), 48.
2. "What Is Authentic Relating?" Authentic Relating Training, accessed June 1, 2023, https://authenticrelating.co/what-is-ar.
3. "About Nonviolent Communication (NVC)," NVC Academy, accessed June 1, 2023, https://nvcacademy.com/nonviolent-communication/about-nonviolent-communication-nvc.
4. Sarah Knight, *The Life-Changing Magic of Not Giving a F*ck: How to Stop Spending Time You Don't Have with People You Don't Like Doing Things You Don't Want to Do* (New York: Little, Brown, 2015).

9. NAME WHAT YOU AUTHENTICALLY VALUE

1. S. Dixon, "Average Daily Time Spent on Social Media Worldwide, 2012–2022," Statista, August 22, 2022, www.statista.com/statistics/433871/daily-social-media-usage-worldwide.

10. CALL IN YOUR RESOURCES

1. Hart Haragutchi, "EFT Tapping (Emotional Freedom Technique)," Choosing Therapy, May 5, 2022, www.choosingtherapy.com/eft-tapping.
2. Wim Hof Method, "Cold Therapy," accessed December 14, 2023, www.wimhofmethod.com/cold-therapy.
3. Kimberly Dawn Neumann, "Red Light Therapy: Benefits, Side Effects, and Uses," *Forbes*, June 27, 2023, www.forbes.com/health/body/red-light-therapy.
4. "Infrared Saunas: What They Do and 6 Health Benefits," Health Essentials, Cleveland Clinic, April 14, 2022, https://health.clevelandclinic.org/infrared-sauna-benefits.
5. M. C. Pascoe and I. E. Bauer, "A Systematic Review of Randomised Control Trials on the Effects of Yoga on Stress Measures and Mood," *Journal of Psychiatric Research* 68 (2015): 270–282.
6. K. T. Laird, I. Vergeer, S. E. Hennelly, and P. Siddarth, "Conscious Dance: Perceived Benefits and Psychological Well-Being of Participants," *Complementary Therapies in Clinical Practice* 44 (July 5, 2021), https://pubmed.ncbi.nlm.nih.gov/34260998.

7. Trauma Prevention Institute, (n.d.),
https://traumaprevention.com.

8. Emily Cronkleton, "10 Breathing Techniques for Stress Relief and
More," Healthline, accessed October 18, 2023,
www.healthline.com/health/breathing-exercise#takeaway.

9. J. L. Oschman, G. Chevalier, and Richard Brown, "The Effects of
Grounding (Earthing) on Inflammation, the Immune Response,
Wound Healing, and Prevention and Treatment of Chronic
Inflammatory and Autoimmune Diseases," *Journal of
Inflammatory Research* 8 (March 24, 2015): 83–96,
www.ncbi.nlm.nih.gov/pmc/articles/PMC4378297.

10. Gary Dorrien, "True Religion, Mystical Unity, and the Disinher-
ited: Howard Thurman and the Black Social Gospel," *American
Journal of Theology and Philosophy 39*, no. 1 (2018),
www.jstor.org/stable/10.5406/amerjtheophil.39.1.0074.

11. "Why Laughing Is Good for You," Cleveland Clinic, November 11,
2022, https://health.clevelandclinic.org/is-laughing-good-for-you.

12. Eric Suni and Nilong Vyas, "How Lack of Sleep Impacts Cognitive
Performance and Focus," Sleep Foundation, April 20, 2023,
www.sleepfoundation.org/sleep-deprivation
/lack-of-sleep-and-cognitive-impairment.

13. National Heart, Lung, and Blood Institute, "What Are Sleep
Deprivation and Deficiency?" accessed June 1, 2023,
www.nhlbi.nih.gov/health/sleep-deprivation.

14. Oregon Health and Science University Center for Women's Health,
"The Benefits of a Healthy Sex Life," accessed May 19, 2023,
www.ohsu.edu/womens-health/benefits-healthy-sex-life.

11. MAP YOUR WAY TO WELL-BEING

1. Paul Davies, "Time's Passage Is Probably an Illusion," *Scientific
American*, October 24, 2014, www.scientificamerican.com/article
/time-s-passage-is-probably-an-illusion/.

2. Centers for Disease Control and Prevention, "Life Expectancy,"
accessed December 3, 2023,
www.cdc.gov/nchs/fastats/life-expectancy.htm.

3. Max-Planck-Gesellschaft, "A Healthy Lifestyle Increases Life

Expectancy by Up to Seven Years," ScienceDaily, accessed December 14, 2023, www.sciencedaily.com/releases/2017/07/170720113710.htm.

12. FITTING OUT

1. Joshua Rosenthal, "To Be Happy, Stop Fitting in and Start Fitting Out," Institute for Integrative Nutrition, March 4, 2021, www.integrativenutrition.com/blog /to-be-happy-stop-fitting-in-and-start-fitting-out.

13. THE POWER OF COMMUNITY

1. Lindsay Lowe, "'Desire Needs Mystery': 75 Best Esther Perel Quotes on Love and Relationships," *Parade*, June 10, 2020, https://parade.com/1049410/lindsaylowe/esther-perel-quotes/.

2. Faith Ozbay, Douglas C. Johnson, Eleni Dimoulas, C. A. Morgan III, Dennis Charney, and Steven Southwick, "Social Support and Resilience to Stress," *Psychiatry* 4, no. 5 (May 2007): 35–40.

ABOUT THE AUTHOR

♡

JOSHUA ROSENTHAL, MScEd, is a pioneer in holistic health, celebrated as the founder of the Institute for Integrative Nutrition (IIN), which has grown into a global community of more than 150,000 students and graduates worldwide. As IIN's director and primary teacher for thirty years, he mentored countless healers and wellness professionals, equipping them with the knowledge and tools to guide others toward integrative wellness.

Joshua's influential work has earned him recognition and features in prominent media outlets such as the *New York Times* and *Forbes*. His transformative books, including *Integrative Nutrition: A Whole-Life Approach to Health and Happiness*, emphasize holistic methods for promoting well-being in all areas of life.

Passionate about philanthropy, Joshua actively engages in global initiatives promoting freedom and empowerment for disadvantaged groups. He also supports startups, including Knew Health, a wellness-focused medical cost-sharing company, and AgelessRx, a platform committed to slowing down aging via practical, innovative approaches.

As a highly sensitive healer with over thirty years of experience in whole foods, coaching, and teaching, Joshua continues to shape the health and wellness landscape, empowering individuals across the globe to embrace a balanced lifestyle that nourishes body, mind, and spirit.